Praise for
Adjust Your Life

There are so many questions about Chiropractic - this intriguing and educational book answers them. Adjust Your Life leads you through a sensible, accurate, and encouraging discussion that is well worth your time!

- Dr. Jenny Bruck
Author of 52 *Vitality Tools*
Host of the popular podcast *For the Health of It*

Adjust Your Life ... *will help those curious about the benefits of Chiropractic care make an informed decision about how to improve their life. I would recommend this book to anyone who may consider Chiropractic, and also to those who already receive life-changing adjustments - both will gain an understanding of how Chiropractic can help the body heal itself.*

- Miranda Otto
Realtor

Well-written, concise, and easy to read, Adjust Your Life *examines the concepts of Chiropractic and the lifestyle it supports. Anyone looking to make a choice about Chiropractic needs to read this.*

- Matt Otto
Test Technician

Matt, Miranda, and their one-year-old daughter Bailey currently receive Chiropractic care. The results seen and felt by Miranda led to the entire family making a commitment to their health.

ADJUST YOUR LIFE

A GUIDE TO CHIROPRACTIC

Justin C. Chase
Stephanie Foisy Mills, D.C., C.C.W.P.

Chase Intellectual, LLC
New Hampshire

A Chase Intellectual, LLC

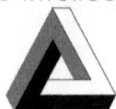

PUBLICATION

Adjust Your Life: A Guide to Chiropractic, First Edition
Justin C. Chase, Stephanie Foisy Mills

Published by:
Chase Intellectual, LLC

Printed by:
Ingram Content Group, Inc.

Editor:
Kate Wiswell

Media/Art Contributions:
Veronica Arabudzki, Veronica Helen Art
Heidi Haavik, Haavik Research

Cover Design:
Gaelyn Larrick, Waking World, Inc.

Website Design:
Tyler Lanning

For product and ordering information, visit:
www.chirocarebook.com

For permission to use material from this text and all other inquiries, please email us at:
support@chirocarebook.com

Chase Intellectual, LLC
PO Box 422
Epsom, NH 03234
United States of America

ISBN 10: 0996778101
ISBN 13: 9780996778107

Dedications

"To my family, for supporting and trusting every decision I make, and to all those pursuing their own health and happiness. I wish you the best."

-Justin C. Chase

"To my dad, for teaching me to think for myself and not just follow the crowd, and to my mom, for being the town crier about Chiropractic. Thank you for discovering the benefits of Chiropractic care and making it a priority for our family. I love you both to the moon and back."

-Dr. Stephanie Foisy Mills

Charitable Contribution

In an effort to promote continued research and education in the Chiropractic profession, a portion of all profits will be donated quarterly to the **Foundation for Vertebral Subluxation**. We believe the Foundation will impact the future of Chiropractic, and we proudly support their mission. Your donations are both accepted, and encouraged. Please donate directly to the Foundation by visiting their website.

Foundation for Vertebral Subluxation
4390 Bells Ferry Road
Kennesaw, Georgia 30144
(404)-247-2550
www.vertebralsubluxation.org

TABLE OF CONTENTS

Adjust Your Life

Appendix – Obtaining Care

Resources

Images and Diagrams

Chapter II.

INTRODUCTION

By Justin C. Chase

I discovered the joys of Chiropractic roughly a year before Dr. Stephanie and I completed this book. I had visited her clinic hoping to find a solution to the back pain I had suffered from for years, but I found much more than that. I found a form of healthcare that was built upon the premise that the human body is remarkable and can heal itself if we take care of it the right way. In working with Dr. Stephanie, I learned that Chiropractic is less about treating symptoms, and more about enabling and promoting the body's innate knowledge – with a little assistance from a chiropractor.

I had initially consider Chiropractic several years before making my first appointment. The stories I had heard about it presented conflicting evidence – some people raved about the benefits of their care, while others condemned the entire profession. These opposing views cast a shadow of doubt in my mind that prevented me from visiting a clinic for years after my initial consideration. Exploring other options and finding no solutions, I finally listened to a close friend's words of advice. I took a "chance" and visited a chiropractor. From the moment I set foot in the office, I knew that Dr. Stephanie and her team would be able to help me. Every team member displayed such confidence and concern for my well-being that I never looked back. I knew that if anyone could help me, it was them.

This book came about as a result of my experiences with Chiropractic. While I recognize that Dr. Stephanie's team may be unique in their talents and demeanor, I didn't want anyone to miss out on the opportunity that Chiropractic presents. I wanted to be sure that people see Chiropractic care for what it is, what it is intended to do, why one might need it, and how they can obtain it. So one day, I simply asked Dr. Stephanie if she had ever considered writing a book – and if she would write one with me. With only a second's hesitation after reading a sample of my work, she agreed to do so. It was the perfect opportunity for her to give back to the profession that has given her so much.

We are happy to present you with this book, written simultaneously by a doctor and a patient. Together, we have worked to expose Chiropractic for what it truly is. We are confident that you, the reader, will be able to make an informed decision about Chiropractic care after you have completed this book. Most importantly, though, we hope that it will help you *Adjust Your Life*, and empower you to make better decisions concerning the treatment of your body.

I.

SETTING THE STAGE

By Justin C. Chase

In order to understand the purpose and function of Chiropractic care, we must first develop a proper perspective. Take a minute to think of a time when you were on a cell phone with a poor connection; how frustrating was it? Did you feel like it was easy to communicate and achieve the purpose of your call?

Now imagine that you are driving to the vacation home of a close friend in rural New Hampshire. You have been driving for hours, and the GPS just stopped working. You haven't seen a road sign you recognize for miles. You have a cell phone and try to call your friend (who still has a landline) in order to obtain directions. The call goes through, but you can tell it is going to be a rough day; service is terrible out here and is only going to get worse while you drive through the deep valleys and endless wooded hills. As you try to explain where you are, you keep having to repeat yourself, and your friend doesn't seem to be hearing things quite as you say them. Is it the signal that is the problem, or are you just not being clear enough with your descriptions? Frustration mounts, and you begin to use shorter words

1

and phrases, hoping your friend will be able to understand you better. This does not, however, make it any easier for him to identify where you are. In fact, the limited information you are now transmitting may even be making it more difficult for him to figure out what you need. Eventually, with much extra work and perseverance, you will reach your destination – exhausted, frustrated, weakened, and likely very stressed. What if this is how your body felt every day?

Can you imagine living through an experience like this on a daily basis? Most of us don't have to imagine; we need only recognize that it is the fight we engage in every day. Every inch of our body needs to communicate with our nervous system and brain in order to function as intended. But this communication is not magical or infallible. We need clear lines of communication in order for our body to function optimally.

Most communication travels from our cells, organs, and extremities to our brain through the spinal cord. When we neglect our spine, we cause interference between our body and our brain. The nearly infinite number of tasks being carried out by the body at any given time are full of requests, commands, and feedback. What happens when we don't receive all of this information? It is like being lost on the back roads of New Hampshire – we struggle to accomplish even the simplest tasks that we normally take for granted. We suffer in many forms: diseases that our body cannot fight with its full strength, bone degeneration, nervous system disorders, increased stress, and chronic pain. This list grows bigger each day we fail to take care of ourselves. Yet we have seen time and again that the body can heal itself. People miraculously recover from being paralyzed, awake from a coma after months, or beat cancer without the use of drugs, radiation, or therapy. A body, however, cannot fight something it does not know exists; communication is key, and the spinal cord is the highway on which this communication travels.

There is a reason our brains are encased in the bones that comprise our skulls. There is also a reason our spinal cords travel through many vertebra, surrounded by a protective layer of bone, tissue, and fluid. The spinal cord is an essential asset, and therefore the structure of the human body is designed to protect it. Unfortunately, we can place demands on our bodies that exceed natural limitations. Deficiencies caused by poor eating habits, physical damage caused by overloading or overworking muscle and bone, and internal stressors from our hectic lifestyles all put our bodies at risk. Instead of protecting our spines, we abuse them on a daily basis and pay little attention, despite the fact that the spine protects one of the most essential pieces of the body.

Chiropractic care deals primarily with identifying and correcting subluxations (or misalignments) in the spine. Your spine not only protects your spinal cord, it also serves as an anchor for many of your muscles and ligaments. Each vertebra (individual bone of the spine) consists of an arch of bone, which creates a tube or tunnel through which the spinal cord runs. Smaller bundles of nerves exit between adjacent vertebrae, creating a connection between the nerve endings found throughout the body, and the brain. When one vertebra is subluxated or out of place, it puts stress on nerve pathways exiting the spine, and/or the spinal cord itself.

What causes subluxations? Though we will talk in much greater depth about this later, it is a combination of physical forces, toxins or chemicals, and stressors. Physical forces can be those caused by trauma like a car accident or fall, but can also be caused by repetitive tasks like carrying a bag or wearing high heels. Chemical changes caused by toxins within the body can influence the ways that our muscles behave – muscles that are intended to work with other body tissues, like tendons and ligaments, in order to keep the spine aligned. Changes in muscle behavior caused by toxins or stress can misalign connected vertebrae. Think about how tight your neck and shoulder muscles end up after a long, stressful week at work; this same tightness is pulling on the spine, and can certainly contribute to subluxations if left unchecked.

The interference in communication caused by the mechanical pressure of subluxations on the nerves of your body can be exemplified by sitting on your hand or foot. After several minutes you may lose feeling in the limb, or feel a tingling sensation. Often, you'll even find it difficult to squeeze your hand, move your fingers or toes, or fully control their functions. Though the way the body responds to pressure on nerve roots and the spinal cord is much more complex, this does serve as an example to assist in your understanding. It demon-strates in a simple form what is happening to your body as nerves struggle to communicate with the brain. Loss of function, feeling, and control result.

In a study by Seth Sharpless (1975), it was found that a pressure on spinal roots as small as 10 mm Hg (millimeters of mercury) – equal to roughly the weight

4

of a dime - can cause a serious disruption in nerve conductivity. In as few as fifteen minutes, this small pressure can cause a 40% reduction in conductivity, and nears 50% after thirty minutes. When this pressure is relieved, normal function often returns within minutes. However, when a more significant pressure is applied, longer term conductivity losses can occur, with nerves failing to regain normal function even after several hours of recovery time.

There are other, more complex factors that contribute to nerve interference - Dr. Stephanie talks about some of these - but to go into detail on this topic is far beyond the intended scope of this book. Regardless, mechanical interferences alone are enough to cause significant disruptions in the transmissions between body and brain.

Wouldn't you notice if your body wasn't communicating with your brain properly? Maybe, but it is not as likely as you may think. When changes happen to our body over time, we rarely notice the effects, whether they are good or bad. We tend to notice visual changes more aptly than internal changes, but even this takes time. For example, people who put on a lot of weight rarely notice the change in their body until they actually weigh themselves or look in a mirror. Do you remember feeling different as a child?

When we look back ten or twenty years, we can certainly say we feel different now than we did then. Do you feel significantly different on a daily basis, though? As you grow one day older, do you notice a deterioration of your cells, speed of thought, or coordination? These changes happen over time, just as your body loses its ability to communicate over time. A loss of as much as 60% of the conductivity of your nerves may not be felt, despite what you may think. Nerves transmit more information than pain or perceptual data – they also relay internal information, send feedback, and receive commands from the brain, among other things. Even a pinched nerve does not always result in pain, though it can cause changes in how the nervous system functions.

The importance of the spine and spinal cord is undebatable. An individual who is paralyzed shows us exactly what happens when our spine suffers severe damage due to an immediate injury. Are you willing to slowly squeeze the life out of yourself by letting your spine suffer each day? There will come a point when the damage can be felt, but the time to act is when you are still functioning. Maintaining a healthy spine is much easier than trying to undo years of damage and disregard.

I understand if you don't believe you are neglecting, damaging, or otherwise hurting your spine. In the same token, I also understand that some teenagers drive fast and do not believe they will ever get in an accident, that some people who smoke do not think it will hurt them, and that people who have cancer often "feel fine" until they are terminal. What we have yet to learn or from experience, we often fail to understand or consider. The purpose of this book is to help you gain perspective, become informed, and then make the decision to seek care or continue as you were.

References

Sharpless, S. K. (1975). Susceptibility of spinal roots to compression block. National Institute of Health, Research Status of Spinal Manipulative Therapy. DHEW Publications 76-998:155.

Additional Resources

Chicken Soup for the Chiropractic Soul by Jack Canfield and Mark Victor Hansen

II.

KNOWLEDGE AND PERCEPTION

Brain and Nervous System 101
By Justin C. Chase

The brain works as the command center of the body, communicating with and controlling it through means of the nervous system. The brain and nervous system are the master coordinators of the body, by which nearly every activity is controlled. Since the brain handles millions of interactions each minute, it is essential that each communication it sends and receives is processed quickly and correctly.

The brain and nervous system communicate through the use of neurons – made up of a cell body, dendrites, and axons. For the purposes of this discussion, dendrites branch off from the cell body and can be likened to the roots of a tree. Dendrites are the receivers of incoming signals. The axons send both chemical and electrical impulses to neighboring nerve cells. Through the use of this wide-ranging system, our entire body can send information to, and receive communication from, the brain.

The nervous system is made up of several key pieces.

It is divided into the Central Nervous System (CNS) and the Peripheral Nervous System (PNS). As you can likely tell, one is centrally contained and the other extends to the rest of the body. The CNS is comprised of the brain and spinal cord, through which sensory and motor information are transferred between the brain and other body parts. Without these communications the brain cannot control the body or receive sensory information.

The Peripheral Nervous System has two major parts: the Autonomic Nervous System (ANS), and the Somatic Nervous System (SNS). The ANS is made of up two systems that are beyond conscious control: the Parasympathetic Nervous System and the Sympathetic Nervous System. These are automatic response systems that react to environmental needs, level of activity, and danger. The ANS is responsible for your breathing, heartbeat, digestion, organ function, etc., all of which are essential to life. The Somatic Nervous System is responsible for controlling movement, speech, and any other conscious behaviors we exhibit. Without the SNS, we would be unable to walk, talk, play catch, or do any other activity involving conscious movement.

The importance of the brain and nervous system (which includes the spinal cord) to everyday function is evidenced in the structure of the body. Both the brain and spinal cord are protected by bone. Since the skull is made up of interlocking cranial bones, it is strong and durable, damaged only by significant blunt force or a piercing blow. One of the common physical dangers to our brain is the danger of concussion, which Dr. Stephanie provides information on in a later chapter. The spine is not like the skull, however. Because it has to be flexible, the spine has weaknesses. Though protected by the vertebrae of our spine, the spinal nerves are at risk when vertebrae shift or move out of place. This can be caused by many things that will be discussed throughout this book, but these shifts (or subluxations) are dangerous to the nervous system and can be very harmful. When subluxations occur, they cause interference in the function and operation of the nervous system – both the Central and Peripheral systems – since much of the body's communication travels through the spinal cord.

In addition to protecting the nervous system, the spine is also a key structural element of our bodies. As previously mentioned, it serves as an anchor for many of the body's structures; the spine supports the head, serves as an attachment point for the ribs and shoulders, and is in turn supported by the pelvis. Without the spine and soft tissue, our body would be unable to support itself, and it would fall apart.

The spine is intended to have a natural curvature, which promotes both range of motion and the ability to bear loads evenly. This natural curve allows the body to distribute weight and stand up to the rigors of life. Much like the design of a bridge, when one area becomes compromised, the whole structure can be at risk. Continued deterioration will lead to the eventual failure of the structure.

The lower back or lumbar should have a curve towards the front of the body (anterior), as it does when you try to stand your straightest and contract your abdomen. As your spine approaches the shoulders and neck, the thoracic curve should reverse the direction as it reaches the more rigid upper back. Your cervical spine (or neck) should have a gentle curve that reflects the lumbar curve. Essentially the forward curve of the lumbar and cervical vertebrae function to bear the weight of the upper body and head, respectively. Contradictions in these curves lead to range of movement problems and the inability to properly distribute and bear weight.

Figure 2.1 and Figure 2.2 below illustrate the ideal curvature of the spine. Note the nerve roots exiting between each vertebra.

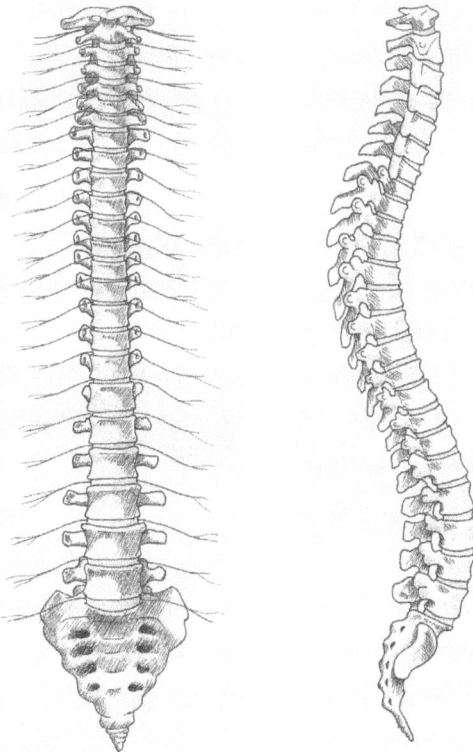

Figure 2.1 (Above left): Posterior/Rear View of Spine
Figure 2.2 (Above right): Lateral/Side View of Spine

Source: Arabudzki, V. H. (2015). Posterior and lateral spine view. Veronica Helen Art, New Hampshire.

Understanding Vertebral Subluxation
By Stephanie Foisy Mills, D.C., C.C.W.P.

The heart of Chiropractic is the detection and correction of the vertebral subluxation. The practice of Chiropractic is an art, science, and philosophy. At the risk of over simplifying, the Chiropractic philosophy is that your body has an innate wisdom, and that subluxation interferes with that. The art is in locating the subluxation and using the best approach, at the right time, to restore normalcy. The science is in understanding the anatomical, neurological and physiological impact of subluxation.

But what exactly is a "subluxation"? Chiropractors have struggled with this question for decades, trying to agree on a definition that takes all aspects into consideration. When Chiropractic was founded in 1895, the term subluxation was originally borrowed from the medical community. The medical definition of a subluxation is often accepted as less than a true dislocation (luxation). However, when subluxation was adopted by the Chiropractic profession, it took on a wider physiological meaning along with a deeper philosophical meaning.

When your spine has a subluxation, it is more than just a bone out of place. It causes detrimental changes in your neurology, musculature, connective tissue, joint function, and more. As science and technology have advanced, we have begun to be able to measure and describe the effects of subluxations and the positive changes that occur through the Chiropractic adjustment.

The scientific understanding is evolving, and as it does it is supporting many of the basic premises in Chiropractic that were established over one hundred years ago. While historical definitions still hold value, new definitions are more relevant, encompassing advances in thought. These new definitions themselves are continuing to evolve, becoming more precise as we better understand the human body. Originally developed by A.E. Homewood, the five component vertebral subluxation complex has been widely utilized in Joseph Flesia, Jr.'s work. It documents five aspects of the Chiropractic lesion:

1. Kinesiopathology: spinal pathomechanics, including alignment and motion irregularities
2. Neuropathology: compressed or facilitated nerve tissue
3. Myopathology: muscle spasm, muscle weakness/atrophy
4. Histopathology: inflammation, edema and swelling of tissue
5. Pathophysiology: adaptive changes such as degeneration, bone spurs, fibrous tissue and/or erosion

(Homewood, 1973; Flesia, 1992)

The five-component model has been expanded upon by other authorities to include connective tissue pathology and vascular abnormalities. Although the definition of subluxation may still be changing with the advancing science, the Chiropractic lesion clearly exists and is a detriment to health.

Proprioception
By Stephanie Foisy Mills, D.C., C.C.W.P.

Though much too complicated to address fully in anything less than an entire book, I want to at least introduce the newest discussions regarding proprioceptive input and its relationship to subluxation and the brain-body function. Movement causes signals to be sent to your brain from structures called mechanoreceptors. These proprioceptive signals are like a "positive body thought," and in a way fuel your brain. These signals are interpreted by your brain in order to determine where your body is in space. They are used in deciding the next command signals to be sent back to your body.

To keep it simple, the lack of movement from a subluxated spinal joint causes abnormal proprioceptive input (information) to be sent to the brain, fitting under the "neuropathology" category of the five component model discussed previously. The brain in turn makes decisions based on faulty information from the body. From there, all heck breaks loose, physiologically speaking! Dr. Heidi Haavik explains how a Chiropractic adjustment can act like a computer re-boot for the brain via its effect on mechanoreceptors in her book, *The Reality Check* (2014). On the next page there are two diagrams from Dr. Haavik's book demonstrating the cycle of abnormal joint movement and dysfunctional processing by the brain (bottom diagram). It also demonstrates the positive effect of a Chiropractic adjustment on brain function (top diagram).

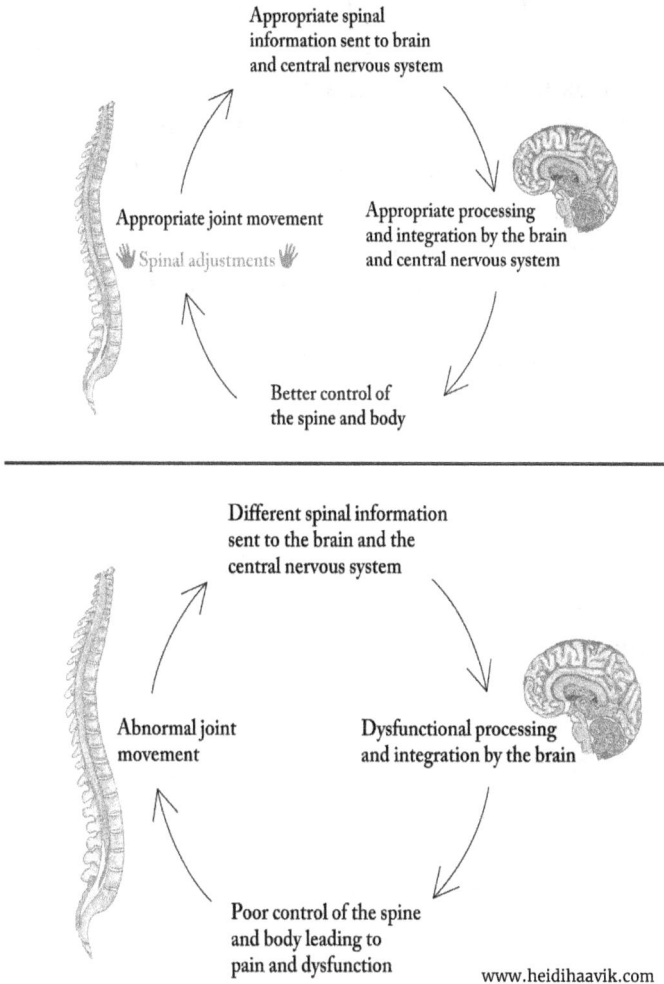

Appropriate spinal information sent to brain and central nervous system

Appropriate joint movement

Spinal adjustments

Appropriate processing and integration by the brain and central nervous system

Better control of the spine and body

Different spinal information sent to the brain and the central nervous system

Abnormal joint movement

Dysfunctional processing and integration by the brain

Poor control of the spine and body leading to pain and dysfunction

www.heidihaavik.com

Figure 2.3: Receiving Adjustments (top) vs. Subluxated (bottom)

Source: Haavik, H. (2014). The reality check: A quest to understand Chiropractic from the inside out. Auckland, New Zealand: Haavik Research Limited, p. 54. Reproduced with permission.

15

While I have discussed some of the scientific explanations of the subluxation itself and its effects, I can't leave this section without also giving the philosophical implications of subluxation a moment of attention. The human body is self-healing, self-organizing, and innately intelligent.

From a vitalistic perspective, subluxation interferes with the body's ability to express its innate intelligence. In short, a subluxated vertebra negatively changes the brain and body's ability to communicate and to keep harmony and balance within its ecosystem. Much of the Chiropractic profession has chosen to disassociate with this philosophy, in order to be more accepted in scientific circles. However, I believe that science alone cannot yet explain the whole mystery of life. I think there is an organization in the universe, a spark of life, and it has an impact on healing and vitality. I just cannot ignore it in the name of science.

Throughout the last century subluxation has been a radical idea; it has revolutionized how we interact with the nervous system and has altered the course of healthcare. Since its inception, people have reported reduced symptoms, normalized body functions, increased energy, elevated mood, improved sleep, and more. Even though we may still not understand fully the complexity of subluxation, there is no doubt that Chiropractic care has positively affected the lives of millions. As one of my practice members said after avoiding Chiropractic for over twenty years, eventually giving it a try in his sixties with remarkable results, "the proof is in the pudding."

Perception and Adaptation
By Stephanie Foisy Mills, D.C., C.C.W.P.

Your body is brilliantly designed to interact with your environment and adapt to it. Your senses do the perceiving: temperature, visual input of the objects around you, smells, tastes, noises... you know the senses! Your brain integrates these messages and formulates a response. On a cold day the hairs on your bare arms stand up with goose bumps. The sudden sound of an animal scampering in the leaves may startle you, causing your eyes to dilate as you look around for danger. Opening a package of chicken that smells fishy churns your stomach, as your brain surmises that the meat has gone bad and could be dangerous to eat. Your nervous system is key to your ability to understand your environment and act appropriately for survival.

This ability to sense what is happening and respond appropriately applies in many ways. Your immune system senses when your body has been invaded by unwanted organisms, communicating this with the nervous system, which coordinates the appropriate response. This correct response is a set of symptoms designed to rid your body of the offender.

Symptoms are not always fun, but they serve an important purpose. One night I had consumed left over Chinese food; it tasted good at the time, but several hours later my stomach began to ache and I found myself vomiting uncontrollably. Was I "sick," or was this actually the perfect response by my body to rid itself of

17

danger? A quick, strong reaction by your nervous system when exposed to a pathogen is, in fact, a fantastic sign of health. The more efficiently your body can rid itself of a bug, the smaller the likelihood a pathogen has of replicating itself and making its way deeper into your body.

The idea of symptoms like vomiting, diarrhea, coughing, stuffy nose or fever as "bad" things is a misunderstanding of the brilliance of your nervous system. Symptoms are an appropriate response to your environment for the protection of your body. But for your body to act appropriately it must first sense what's going on, interpret it, and act accordingly. Having a spine that is free from the stress of subluxations can improve the function of your nervous system and its ability to accurately interpret your environment and respond to it. These responses are essential to your survival – so it is vital that the body is able to communicate effectively and efficiently.

Addressing Concerns
By Justin C. Chase

You will be exposed primarily to the good that Chiropractic appears to be correlated with; what about the bad, you may ask? The truth is, there is very little. Of course there are some websites that dispute what Chiropractic has done, where contributors claim to have suffered injuries. It is very possible that these injuries are real; accidents happen in every medical profession. But, injuries in Chiropractic are few and far between, caused most often by lapses in technique rather than by any flaw in the theory.

From the people who dispute the underlying principles of Chiropractic (often members of other medical practices and the drug industry), what proof have we heard about the dangers of Chiropractic? If there were any proof, it would surely be at the forefront of the argument. Some people say Chiropractic is dangerous, that it doesn't work, and that everyone should avoid Chiropractic care. But means of evaluation, such as x-rays, show that it does work. Chiropractors help the body regain its natural structure and posture by facilitating the necessary movements of bone and joints. What follows comes solely from the body: there is a correlation between Chiropractic care and the ability of the body to heal itself – and this correlation is much stronger than any that relates Chiropractic to injury or harm.

There have been Doctors of Chiropractic who have written books about the dangers of Chiropractic. Of course, there are dangers to *any* medical practice, particularly those that require years to learn. However, many of these same alarmists are still practicing chiropractors, which casts great doubt over the sincerity of their arguments.

There has been not nearly enough evidence to raise concern over the methods or practices used by chiropractors. Try comparing the malpractice rates of chiropractors with those of medical doctors, surgeons, etc. Despite millions of people receiving Chiropractic adjustments daily, when was the last time you heard about an injury in the news?

The truth is, most arguments against Chiropractic are that it only makes you feel better, that it doesn't actually help, or that it is "all in your head." I understand the idea of a placebo, and it is difficult, if not impossible, to research Chiropractic with a control group and placebo since care involves physically touching patients. It could be hypothesized that even if patients weren't receiving adjustments, the physical sensation of someone else touching their body could have an effect in their mind. Despite these concerns, we have already discussed the proof related to the ability of a chiropractor to properly realign the spine. My question for you, though, is this: "Isn't it enough to feel better?"

It seems that most people come to see a chiropractor because they have pain or discomfort throughout their body. Isn't the goal usually to feel better? To be able to do things you are currently unable to do? A placebo is used in most studies so as not to confuse the effects of a drug or treatment with the effects of the mind. But Chiropractic is based on the premise that the human body does the healing. The power of the mind and the body are precisely what *should* be doing the healing. So when someone asks you, "Do you feel better?" you hope to respond with a resounding "YES!" If there is a common theme between receiving Chiropractic care and feeling better, which it appears by nearly all accounts that there is, what are you waiting for? If you have concerns or questions, see your local chiropractor. If all else fails, reach out to the Chiropractic community at large, or contact us. I think as you continue reading this book that any underlying fears you have will be relieved.

References

Flesia, J. M. (1992, March). The vertebral subluxation complex: An integrative perspective. International Review of Chiropractic, 25-27.

Haavik, H. (2014). The reality check: A quest to understand Chiropractic from the inside out. Auckland, New Zealand: Haavik Research Limited.

Homewood, A. E. (1973). The neurodynamics of the vertebral subluxation (2nd ed.). Canada: Chiropractic Publishers.

Additional Resources

The 14 Foundational Premises for Scientific and Philosophical Validation of the Chiropractic Wellness Paradigm by James L. Chestnut
The Reality Check by Heidi Haavik

III.

THE MAKING OF A CHIROPRACTOR

By Stephanie Foisy Mills, D.C., C.C.W.P.

Though I didn't realize it at the time, Chiropractic chose me when I was very young. As a child, I made monthly visits to an old-time New England chiropractor with my parents. Initially I would just tag along and watch in amusement as my parents each mounted a noisy table, were pushed on in some sort of pattern, and then arose with joyful smiles and improved gaits.

One afternoon the doctor asked my mother's permission to check my spine; he knew I had been suffering from ear infections for years, and that the recent installation of surgical tubes hadn't resolved them. I was apprehensive about my first spinal alignment, but it wasn't long before having my turn on the table became the routine. I remember leaving his office feeling a sense of relaxation, while somehow feeling more energetic and alive at the same time. I liked it, even though I couldn't articulate why.

I didn't notice that I wasn't getting sick as often as I used to, nor did I notice that my usual earaches were no longer a bother. Sometimes it's harder to notice what is not happening. When things get better, we often forget that there was ever a problem. Many years later, as a young adult, I finally connected the dots: my chronic ear infections had become less frequent once I began getting adjusted.

With this newly realized connection, I decided that I wanted to help people like my parents alleviate their back pain naturally, and help kids like myself resolve their ear aches and infections. When I arrived at Palmer College of Chiropractic in Davenport, Iowa at the age of twenty, I was surprised to find that most other students had their own Chiropractic story of some similar variation.

There were quite a few former athletes who had recovered from injuries with the help of a chiropractor, and a handful of other young students felt Chiropractic care had helped them overcome childhood illnesses like my own. There were also those who were arriving for their second career in life; men and women in their thirties, forties, and even fifties, willing to leave their comfortable lives, relocate their families to Iowa, endure thousands of hours of schooling and take huge educational debt, all in order to "give back" to a profession for helping them restore their own health.

However, the most interesting group of students to me was the second- and third-generation chiropractors-to-be. They had lived differently than the rest of us, and had a unique way of looking at life. I spent many nights discussing, inquiring, and listening to the wisdom that had been handed down to these special students from their parents and grandparents. Looking back, most of us appeared to have been called to Chiropractic with a greater purpose. We didn't choose it, it chose us.

I had entered Chiropractic College thinking I would learn to help people solve their aches, pains, and chronic problems. But in actuality I left with a much broader understanding. I spent four thousand hours at University learning the intricate details of cellular function at the biochemical level, about organ physiology, microbiology, and human pathologies.

By the end of my education, I understood that health comes from within. It comes from taking good care of your body, by giving it all of what it needs and none of what it doesn't. The biggest "a-ha!" moment: realizing that each of us has a wisdom in our body. It is an inner intelligence that knows how to digest an apple and turn it into new cells, an inborn intelligence that knows how fast to make our heart beat, and how to heal our skin when we get a paper cut. We have a wisdom that acts to preserve our body in all circumstances, and if we would recognize it and honor it, we would all be better off.

Though my perspective changed as I learned more about the intricacies and capabilities of the human body, not every chiropractor leaves graduation a changed person. Many continue to see the Chiropractic adjustment as a modality, as a pain reliever for low back and neck pain. These philosophical differences have created a wide divide within the profession. While each licensed chiropractor you may meet has a degree in Chiropractic, the vast majority will differ greatly in practice.

Chiropractic is a science, an art, and a philosophy. Just as no two artists will create identical paintings and no two philosophers will see life through quite the same lens, every chiropractor will approach their art in their own unique style. As you come to a better understanding of the science of Chiropractic, you will be able to choose your practitioner wisely. You will begin to understand what you need, and will be able to find a practitioner who supports that.

Structure dictates function, in life as well as in your body. Without proper structure, there can't be optimal function. That is the gem within Chiropractic – chiropractors create the best possible alignment of the bones that protect your brain and nervous system, allowing your master system to orchestrate and animate your body toward reaching its fullest potential.

IV.
SENSE OF DIRECTION

By Justin C. Chase

Prior to making a commitment to any form of health care, exercise regimen, or diet, you must determine what your long-term goals are. Without doing so, you will be unable to make value judgements on the different options you encounter. In order to ensure that each decision you make will help you over the course of your life, a sense of direction is essential.

What are your ultimate goals? Only after you have answered this question can you truly begin to progress towards health and happiness. Looking only to your immediate health is not sustainable – a decision you make today may relieve pain or suffering temporarily, but carry long term consequences that counteract any immediate benefits.

What goals do you have, and how can they be defined? If you are like most people, you have likely tried some sort of exercise program, fad diet, or miracle remedy that turned out to be quackery. It is also likely that you didn't stick with the diet, you stopped working out, or you decided to try some other remedy you saw on TV. It has happened to us all.

There are several problems with this approach. I imagine you had some short term goal, such as losing fifty pounds or lowering your blood pressure so your doctor would let you go back to eating junk food. Maybe you didn't put in your full effort one hundred percent of the time, or research what you were doing thoroughly enough. These are all results of looking only at the immediate. When your goals are aimed primarily at the present they can be difficult to maintain, particularly if you do not see immediate changes. Realize that it has taken a lifetime for your health to deteriorate, and it cannot be recovered in a day.

In order to think long term, you need to consider the aspects of your life that truly make you happy. What makes you happy is likely very different from what makes your neighbor or colleague happy – and that is okay. In addition to your happiness, you should determine what is required in your life. Consider the requirements of your job, such as driving for long periods, lifting, twisting, working odd hours, etc. Also consider the capabilities necessary to pursue hobbies, take care of your children, and perform day-to-day tasks. You need to be able to perform necessary tasks without causing injury or overt discomfort in order to achieve overall health and happiness.

What is it, then, that truly makes you happy? Is it going for a long run on a warm summer morning, or playing with your grandchildren in the backyard? Would being able to read a book without hurting your neck make you happy? Perhaps you'd like to be free of sickness and avoid making the same frequent doctor visits you've made every year of your life. Do you want to be able to go camping with your family and wake up feeling energized rather than lethargic? Or do you simply want to be free of aches and pains? The question is yours to answer. Whatever you decide will make you happy, improve your quality of life, or help you perform household tasks with greater comfort is certainly worth pursuing.

In addition to your physical comforts, what future ambitions do you have concerning your work or hobbies? In my experience as an educator, I have worked with people ranging in age from about eight years old to eighty. The happiest people I encounter are not those with the most money, the largest collection of possessions, or those with the most friends... the happiest people I have met are the ones who have a purpose in life. If you aren't learning new things or working towards a future ambition, it is very easy to become stagnant. Not only in your work life, but in your personal life as well.

Anyone who has become complacent will find it difficult to make health changes, since that requires a commitment that may be abnormal for their way of life. If you are one of those people, I implore you to consider ways in which you can advance yourself in the workplace or by finding and experimenting with a new hobby. What can you learn, build, do, or experience? Constant growth is essential to living a happy and fulfilling life. Explore these options, because they will give purpose to your life and make your health goals worth pursuing. When you have something to live for, the quality of your life shifts from an afterthought to the forefront of your consciousness.

28

As you continue to read and progress through this book, reflect back on these goals often. It is okay to modify them as your vision of what your life could be becomes clearer. Your goals should be constructed and realized over a period of time, not in a matter of minutes. By putting significant thought into them, you can be sure they truly reflect your innermost motives. This means that they are important to you. It is likely that your goals contain some of the most important pieces of your life, such as your children, grandchildren and family, your work, your favorite hobbies, or your biggest problems and concerns that need to be overcome. The more important these things are to you, the more consistent you will be in working towards them - because failure is simply not an option.

What does this discussion have to do with health care choices and Chiropractic care? Do some research on the prescriptions and over the counter medicines you use, then try to determine the side-effects of these products. Many people intentionally avoid doing this. I'll let you in on a secret: not reading the side-effects of the medication you are taking does not mean that these side effects do not exist. Avoiding the truth is going to cause you to fail in almost every endeavor you decide to pursue. You should acknowledge that medication is not an end-all-be-all-fix-all. It is, in many cases, a shortcut leading to immediate relief of symptoms- a shortcut that can lead to long term dependency and greater problems. It is the type of shortcut that can get you lost in the woods, with no clear way out.

Even if you have not formulated all of your goals yet, think about the ones you currently have in mind. How many of them involve taking drugs?

If your goals *don't* include relying on medication, your healthcare options become limited. Your focus must then shift to prevention. Simple exercise and nutrition changes can help prevent many of the issues that medications are prescribed to "fix". But what if I told you there was something that could complement exercise and nutrition? Something that could surround you with an environment focusing on health, improve your body's internal communication, and ensure that your mind and body are performing at peak levels? I hope that you've made the connection – I've already told you about it. Chiropractic care is a way to make exercise and nutrition more effective for your body, and improve the internal communication of your central nervous system, helping to limit your need for medication or surgery.

If your goal is to achieve health of the mind and body, Chiropractic can help. Consider the nearly infinite number of processes being performed by your body in any given moment. Are you consciously breathing? Are you making your heart beat, drawing in oxygen from the air into your lungs, and then sending it through the body by means of your blood? Are you fighting infections, replacing worn out cells, and making all the connections required to do the things you take for granted, such as seeing, hearing, and thinking?

Your body is capable of incredible things. Imagine how much more capable it can be if it is communicating as it was designed to, as opposed to losing data like your cell phone with a poor connection! If you can imagine this, you can make it a reality. But you can't do it alone. I am confident that as you continue your journey into the world of Chiropractic, you will begin to see what I see. I ask only that you approach this book with an objective mind. Don't believe what we tell you simply because we have put it in print – instead read it, analyze it, and make your own determinations of what you believe. In this way, you can be confident that you are making an informed decision concerning how you treat your body and view Chiropractic care.

Realize, however, that Chiropractic care is not the easy way out. It is not to be used as a substitute for hard work, planning, and action. It is a complement to a balanced and well thought-out lifestyle approach. Which means: it is a tool to be used as you strive to reach your ultimate health goals.

V.
HEALTHY LIFESTYLES

By Stephanie Foisy Mills, D.C., C.C.W.P.

Chiropractic care does not consist of nutrition, exercise, or mental management. Chiropractic focuses on the correction of subluxations in order to reduce stress on the nervous system. This allows the body to fully express itself. However, most patients find that their chiropractors are extremely knowledgeable and often passionate about fitness and nutrition. Chiropractors encourage patients to take action towards better lifestyle choices because we know that small changes can add up to a life changing sum. We encourage you to educate yourself, make better choices, and set goals. The bottom line is that Chiropractic adjustments set the stage for healing, but the basic needs for cellular function can't be overlooked. The health equation is pretty simple. First, give your cells the required raw materials to work with, and second, protect them from toxins and poisons.

Fuel
While I could write volumes on food alone, my purpose here is to get you thinking, asking questions, and broadening your perspective. Food is your body's

fuel. It gives you energy, provides the building blocks for your body to make new cells, and provides vitamins which are crucial pieces of many important body functions. For a moment, think of your body as an exotic sports car. After all, the human body is one the finest creations on the planet. What grade of gasoline are you willing to put in the tank of your prized sports car? Of course, you want the highest quality to ensure peak performance. Now, consider what octane foods you are currently fueling your body with. Are you eating "high test" foods, or are you buying the cheap stuff? Are you taking care of your most prized possession (your body), or are you neglecting it, resulting in a buildup of body sludge?

The nutritional quality of your food matters. Foods that are whole (not processed) and fresh are the most nutritious. But this is just scratching the surface! Avoiding foods that nature never intended us to eat is important as well. Genetically, we are meant to be "hunter-gatherers." Our genes are the same as our Paleolithic ancestors, yet our modern diet is vastly different. Our hunter-gatherer genes are doing the best they can to help us adapt to our present day diet, but eating unnatural food is slowly killing us. Seven of the top ten causes of death in America are chronic disease- related (Deaths and Mortality, 2015). These illnesses are primarily a result of our lifestyle. They are diseases that creep up on us slowly, caused by poor food choices, sedentary living, and toxic exposures. Diseases like diabetes, heart disease, cancer, and dementia - the direct results of decisions that we make every day over the course of many years.

The best way to minimize your risk for chronic disease is to adapt a way of eating that is best suited for your body. I encourage everyone to take steps towards "eating like a caveman." In short, this means eating things that grew from the ground or walked upon it. Eat plenty of fruits, veggies, nuts, and seeds. Eat protein from animals that were allowed to live the way that they were meant to live. For example, choose to eat cows that were allowed to walk around and eat grass, instead of those that were corn-fed and lived in crowded and unsanitary feed lots, choose fish that swam and ate in the wild as opposed to farm-raised fish, and eat wild game meats, too.

Whenever possible, avoid eating animals that were kept in contained lots. Also avoid soy, dairy products, added sugars, wheat, grains, gluten, and corn. This may be shocking and contrary to what you've learned in the past, but you will have less inflammation, fewer digestive problems, and more energy if you eat like a hunter-gatherer. For more on this, check out any Paleo cookbook, blog, or social media site. You can, of course, also consult your doctor for his specific nutritional recommendations.

For some, the idea of "giving up" favorite foods or beverages becomes paralyzing. We might throw our hands up in the air and say, "I can't do all that, so why bother?" The idea isn't to overhaul your eating habits overnight. It is to make small manageable changes that don't cause you to stress, feel deprived, or unhappy. As a place to begin, add one healthy item to each meal. Eat your healthy item first. For example, eat an apple for breakfast before your morning bagel. Always drink a full glass of water before drinking that *other* beverage. At lunch, start with a salad before your cheeseburger and fries. As you progress, start letting things go. For instance, order your burger without the bun or with a side of veggies instead of fries. As you improve your habits, you'll be feeling less sluggish and more energetic. This will make it easier to continue making changes. Each day, strive to do better than yesterday. If you can achieve this every day (or even most of the time), you will see significant positive changes over long periods of time.

Before leaving this delicious discussion, allow me to remind you that food, even the healthier choices, can be a major source of toxins! Spending a few extra dollars to buy organic produce decreases your exposure to toxic pesticides and herbicides. Don't be afraid of organic, there is no sacrifice in terms of taste (if anything, they taste better!). Try to avoid boxed goods with food additives, preservatives, colors, chemicals, and artificial sweeteners. Furthermore, avoid Genetically Modified foods. GMO stands for Genetically Modified Organism. The ones to watch out for are those that have been modified to be drug/disease resistant. These products have been banned in many other countries because of the potential risks associated with them. Unfortunately, GMO's are not required to be labeled as such in the United States, so buying Certified Organic remains the best bet to avoid them.

You may find that each doctor you talk to has his or her own views on nutrition. There are many differing perspectives on what constitutes "healthy" food, as well as ideas on how to approach diet and overall nutrition.

There are, however, some universal truths: eat a variety of (real) foods, eat more fresh fruit and vegetables (but not too much), and ingest fewer toxins and chemicals by eating organic and avoiding processed food whenever possible. Most of us have a pretty good feel for what foods should be considered healthy, even if we have chosen not to eat them in the past. Read up on nutrition, and be sure to include the Paleo Diet in this reading – then make your own decisions, or consult your doctor, chiropractor, or nutritionist for help.

Oxygen

It seems elementary to say, but our cells need oxygen. As a whole, we have become shallow breathers with poor posture. This lack of oxygen leaves our bodies functioning at a less than optimum level. Incorporate deep breathing exercises, aerobic activities, and/or yoga into your daily routine. Yoga is a fantastic way to improve your breathing, relax your mind, and increase your flexibility. Why not grab a friend and try a class?

We want to breathe the cleanest air possible. Although we have limited control over smog and general pollutants in our environment, we can take action in our homes to improve air quality and limit toxins. For example, when planning to paint or redecorate, try to do it in a season where you can leave windows open all day and all evening. New carpet, new mattresses, fresh paint, etc. will all "off gas." This means that chemical gases are emitted by products in the highest concentrations when they are new. Think new car smell here.

Make your best effort to ventilate areas with new

furniture, or if you are really zealous, buy specialized products like non-toxic wool rugs and organic mattresses and pillows. In addition, keep a generous array of house plants like aloe vera, peace lilies, English ivy, and spider plants. House plants like these have been shown to improve indoor air quality. Indoor air purifying devices are great to help deal with mold and other allergen issues as well.

Water

Our beverage of choice should be water. After being weaned from our mother's breast, water is the only liquid required by our bodies. Why stress your system with a sugary or chemical-laden beverage? Clean, pure water not only satisfies thirst but gives life to our body. Water is important for all functions in the body, including, but not limited to: digestion, toxin and waste removal, and our cooling system (sweat).

How much water should you drink? It seems like an easy question, but experts have had difficulty agreeing on a number. In general you should drink a half an ounce to an ounce of water for every pound you weigh. For example, if you weigh 150 pounds you should drink between 75 and 150 ounces daily. Although this may seem high, many people drink 4-5 cups (or 32-40 ounces) of water regularly, but also drink several cups of milk, soda, and juice daily. If water were substituted in for these other beverages, most people could easily manage to drink the recommended amounts of water. It sounds like a lot of water - and it should, since our body weight is constituted of well over 50% water weight.

The amount your body requires will vary upon the

climate you live in and how much you exercise. One rough way to estimate whether you are drinking enough water is to observe the color of your urine. An ideal color, indicating proper hydration, is a pale yellow or a lemonade color. Of course, watch your urine stream and not the resulting color when mixed with the water in your toilet. Keep in mind that there are other issues that can darken the color of urine, such as vitamins, supplements, or health conditions which require medical attention. If you prefer not to look at your pee, there is another method you can use, though it is considered less reliable. Do a search for "dehydration skin test" online and you can find information on a quick and easy test you can do by pinching the skin on the back of your wrist and watching how quickly it returns to place.

In addition to staying hydrated, be mindful of your water source. City water is often treated with chlorine and chloramine, and may also be fluoridated. If you are lucky enough to have well water, you should have it tested regularly for contaminants since it is not monitored by anyone but you. If you fail to test it, contaminants in your water could be influencing your body. Research water filtration systems like reverse osmosis and carbon filters for your household drinking water and bathing water if necessary. In addition, consider drinking from a glass container instead of plastic. Don't allow one of the most essential ingredients for life to become a daily poison for your body.

Movement

Our Paleolithic ancestors walked approximately nine

miles per day. Movement was a part of life. They hunted and gathered, cared for their young, and built shelter. Nothing was accomplished by sitting around. We humans are designed to move... a lot. As a society, we've lost touch with that fact.

In recent decades, our culture has made a shift in thinking; exercise is now viewed as a means to improve health. This is a good start, but it falls short. Our allopathic research approach has caused us to examine movement requirements by asking, "What is the smallest dosage (amount of exercise) that needs to be given in order to affect a measurable change?" The answer has historically been the age-old mantra of thirty minutes per day, three days per week. But the better question to ask would be, "How much exercise do I need to satisfy my body's biological need for movement?" If we were asking that question, I am confident that we would draw an entirely different conclusion.

Movement has been shown to lessen stress, improve moods, advance learning, and lessen the risk for cancer, heart disease, diabetes, obesity, and depression. Sedentary living has been correlated to an increased risk for death, plain and simple. The moral of the story is to move, and to do it frequently. Move every day, as much as possible! Move in different ways that raise your heart rate, help build muscle, and in ways that improve your flexibility, balance, coordination, and speed. If you need help, find a trainer to construct a program for you that includes aerobic and anaerobic exercises, strength training and flexibility. Not only will this assist you in improving your health, it will increase your confidence and capability to do those things in life that you love.

Sleep

Catching your zzz's is vital to healing, growth, and cell repair. Good sleep and good health go hand-in-hand. There is no doubt that a lack of sleep or an inability to get quality sleep is a significant stressor for your body. If you are having issues with your sleep patterns, first assess your sleep habits. Are you going to bed at the same time each night? Do you have a routine time that you wake, every day? A consistent schedule, even on weekends, is important. Try not to vary it by more than an hour on either end.

Your cells require a certain amount of sleep, and that perfect amount is unique to you. Experts have a range in opinion, but likely between seven and nine hours of sleep for an adult is appropriate, while children need more due to their near-constant growth. Make a goal to clear your schedule to allow for the average eight hours of sleep each night.

As you institute Chiropractic care along with the other lifestyle changes in this chapter and book, it is likely that your sleep will improve on its own. But if you are still having issues, try avoiding screen time a full hour before bed. This means turning off your television, computer, and mobile screens and finding something to do that is not emitting blue light into your eyes. Artificial blue light from electronics can disrupt your natural sleep-wake cycle. You may also need to examine your caffeine use. Afternoon coffee, tea, or soda pop could still be affecting you at bedtime as you try to unwind and fall asleep.

Mental Management

Emotional stress causes stress hormone secretion. Stress hormones cause an alarm state within the body. This alarm state is for our short-term survival. Imagine one of our caveman ancestors. If caveman Bob were out gathering food and unexpectedly came face to face with a lion, Bob would become suddenly alarmed. In fact, Bob's body would go into a "fight or flight" state. Bob would have the choice to fight off the lion, or flee for survival. Either way, his body would benefit from a sympathetic nervous system (stress) response. In this state, Bob's blood pressure would rise, blood would be shunted away from his organs and re-directed to his skeletal muscles, and his mental attention would change. Bob's body would even increase the blood clotting ability of his blood, just in case he was to get cut or injured. All of these changes are meant to be short-term survival techniques. Once the danger has passed, the nervous system returns to its resting, parasympathetic state. Again, the stress state is meant to be short term, to help us deal with immediate danger.

Compare the stress of facing a wild animal to the stress of the modern world. Often times we are mentally stressed for hours or days at a time, causing the same fight or flight stress response to happen within our bodies. But in the modern world, we don't quickly fight or flee the situation; instead we stay stressed for long periods of time. This is extremely taxing on our body, and can contribute to chronic disease. Just look back at the example of Bob in the above paragraph. Note his elevated blood pressure and increased blood clotting ability, both of which are contributors to heart attack and stroke.

In a study published in the European Heart Journal: Acute Cardiovascular Care entitled *Triggering of Acute Coronary Occlusion by Episodes of Anger*, the risk of a heart attack was over eight times higher for the two hour period following an intense bout of anger. Further, heart attack risk was more than nine times higher after an episode of extreme anxiety (Buckley, et al., 2015). Clearly, part of a healthy lifestyle is learning to recognize stressors, and deal with them appropriately so our body can return to its natural state.

There are thousands of books about the health topics I just touched on. I hope at this point to have piqued your interest, so that you can look into them further and come to your own conclusions. Our bodies are very complex, and as such can be difficult to understand. What we know about the human body and how it works should be taken advantage of; we have more knowledge than ever before, even if most of us choose to ignore it. Use your resources, including your doctors, chiropractor, trainer, and the vast network of literature that is available. But, be sure to think for yourself on these topics, and ascertain whether the authors thoughts fit with the purposes of the human body and enable it, rather than handicap it.

References

Buckley, T., Fethney, J., Hanson, P. S., Shaw, E., Tofler, G. H., & Y Soo Hoo, S. (2015). Triggering of Acute Coronary Occlusion by episodes of anger. European Heart Journal: Acute Cardiovascular Care, 1-6.

Deaths and Mortality. (2015, January 20). Retrieved from Centers for Disease Control and Prevention: http://www.cdc.gov/nchs/fastats/deaths.htm

Additional Resources

Everyday Paleo by Sarah Fragoso and Robb Wolf
Food, Inc. directed by Robert Kenner
Impossible Cure: The Promise of Homeopathy by Amy L. Lansky
Love Your Body: Your Path to Transformation, Health, and Healing by N. D. Barry Taylor
National Vaccine Information Center
　　http://www.nvic.org/
Robb Wolf's What is the Paleo Diet?
　　http://robbwolf.com/what-is-the-paleo-diet/
Seeds of Deception: Exposing Industry and Government Lies About the Safety of the Genetically Engineered Foods You're Eating by Jeffrey M. Smith
The Beautiful Truth: The World's Simplest Cure for Cancer directed by Steve Kroschel
The Wellness and Prevention Paradigm by James L. Chestnut

VI.
"WHY ME?"

By Justin C. Chase

"Why me?" This question often comes up when Chiropractic care is mentioned. We make the assumption that because we don't have severe back pain, or have never had a high speed car accident that we don't need Chiropractic care. Unfortunately, bad habits accumulate into a lifetime of small-scale traumatic events, which compound into many of the aches and pains we experience on a daily basis. These events, left unchecked, can interfere with the natural functions of our body and with the communication between our nervous system and brain.

The next time you go to the store or walk down the street, observe the people around you. How many of them have correct posture? How many have the proper neck curvature described and illustrated earlier? It is likely that most of the people you see are carrying weight unevenly, looking down at their cellphone, have their shoulders and back hunched over, or are committing some other form of treason against their body. Our daily lifestyle influences this posture. The way we live our lives has a major impact on how our muscles act and how they influence our skeletal structure. It also determines the benefits (or consequences) of our posture.

Man's lifestyle has evolved significantly since the beginning of the Industrial Age, and that has certainly taken its toll on our bodies. Before the division of labor became prominent, most families grew or raised at least a portion of their own food. This required daily physical activity in order to take care of the needs around the house. Today, the majority of us work jobs that require minimal physical activity. We work on computers, drive cars, and often cut corners where physical activity is an option; we take the elevator instead of the stairs, or take the bus to work instead of walking.

Though we now have access to things that our predecessors would never have dreamed of, our lifestyle has changed the way we use our bodies. Instead of spending the day moving and working to ensure survival, we spend large portions of our time pushing buttons or staring blankly at television sets.

During my first meeting with Dr. Stephanie, she mentioned a theory of hers that was very intriguing to me. She talked about how thousands of years ago, humans spent the majority of their time hunting and gathering food. Their lives depended upon their ability to perform these tasks adequately. This required that humans be physically fit – strong, fast, and durable. Spending most of the day moving around certainly has its benefits. It makes the body strong and lean, and it also helps to keep the entire skeletal structure of the body limber.

Dr. Stephanie explained that while today we spend many hours each day looking down at our computers, cell phones, and other devices, our ancestors likely spent much of their time looking up. They needed to be observant of the world around them. Even while picking fruits and berries or gathering materials for shelter, humans needed constant awareness of their surroundings, which would have required their heads to be lifted.

The neck is not meant to be protruding forward and down all the time. Perhaps in the future our individual vertebra will become larger and more resistant to decay, and the muscles of our neck and spine will do a better job of supporting a forward hung head – but currently, they are not and do not. We are not meant to be looking downwards for most of the day. Our basic functions and body structure are designed for a being that is frequently active. When we do not use our bodies as they are meant to be used, our muscles atrophy. This means that they reduce in size, strength, and capability, further increasing the risk of subluxations as the bones of the spine receive less support from the muscles around them. Our often-inactive lifestyle is a major factor in the need for Chiropractic care, and is one of the many reasons that we repeatedly stress the benefits of exercise and nutrition.

As you consider Chiropractic care, you should look at the things you do as part of your daily routine. Many of these things are detrimental to your health. We often overlook the small aspects of our lives that become habitual, but these little things can quickly become big problems. The wallet that you keep in your back pocket when sitting can exert pressure on your lower back and hips. The oversize purse that you carry on the same shoulder every day can affect the bones in your neck, as your muscles strain to carry the weight evenly. Driving with only one hand on the steering wheel can cause similar problems. Any position that causes the body to be uneven, or to carry weight with an unequal distribution can cause significant problems when it is part of a routine. Even when we do distribute weight evenly, we still need to be careful; activities such as carrying a heavy backpack, moving heavy boxes, or frequent lifting or twisting while bearing weight can all be problematic.

The types of furniture in your home can also be contributing to subluxations. Most couches slant backwards, encouraging you to 'lounge' or lean back. While this is a comfortable position, and it feels great to figuratively "take a load off", there are several problems with most couches.

First, we often use couches to watch television. So, while you lounge back on the couch, your head and neck usually have to be angled forward and down in order to see the TV. This causes the neck to bear the extended weight of the head, which is significantly greater the further forward it extends.

The second problem is that lounging back on the couch disengages most of your core muscles. This leaves the spine essentially unsupported. The natural curve that our spine is supposed to have loses its desired curvature as the core muscles relax, causing it to straighten or even curve in the wrong direction.

The last major problem is that lounging on a couch

means that you are not being active or engaged. Time spent on the couch is a contributing factor to the obesity experienced by many people today. Where our ancestors would spend their evenings outdoors taking care of their animals or performing other chores, we sit and do nothing. This results in burning fewer calories and being less productive. If you simply *have* to sit down, at least go through the effort of finding furniture that is comfortable, but still engages your core muscles.

––––––––––

The way we use technology can have a drastic effect on our bodies. As I mentioned earlier, using a computer all day encourages us to sit in a "comfortable" chair. Comfortable often means relaxed, leading to many of the same issues associated with couches. Most people work eight hours or longer at a time, with just a few short breaks. Eight hours of continuous sitting can wreak havoc on the spine, particularly if workers are not paying attention to their posture.

An emerging fad to counteract this is the idea of a "standing" workstation, which allows workers to set their equipment on a higher surface and stand while working. This encourages them to remain active throughout the day, and keep their core muscles engaged. It also helps prevent workers from looking down at a computer screen – monitors can be set higher on a standing workstation to help maintain posture.

The cell phones we rely so heavily on can also cause problems. "Text Neck", a term coined by Dean Fishman, D.C., is becoming a major problem. Many adolescents, teenagers, and recently many adults, spend significant amounts of time hunched over their phones, browsing the internet, playing games, or texting their friends. This posture continues the trend of our generation, once again causing us to look down with our heads pushed forward. Our bodies are not designed for this.

Another problem with cell phone usage is that when we talk on the phone or text, we regularly use the same hand for these tasks, or worse – hold the phone to our shoulder by craning our necks! The act of holding our phone to our heads or out in front of us with the same hand causes the muscles to act differently on the two sides of our bodies. Habitual phone use in this fashion can cause the muscles to overcompensate and tighten, trying to hold the spine in alignment despite the actions we take against it.

It is likely at this point that you've already begun to identify some aspects of your own life that are negatively influencing your posture, and thus, your spine. That is great! But we haven't even talked about large-scale traumatic incidents yet.

It should be evident that by paying little attention to our posture, we have been doing a lot more harm than good. As we start covering traumatic incidents like car accidents, falls on ice, or broken bones, the concerns start to grow even more rapidly. When we are involved in an accident, even very low-speed collisions can cause whiplash. This is the result of a rapid or abrupt acceleration of the head forward or backwards, and can wreak havoc on the muscles, ligaments, vertebrae, and nerves contained in and around the neck. It can also cause damage to the brain, in the form of a concussion. An incident involving whiplash is highly likely to cause or negatively contribute to subluxations in the spine.

Other aspects of a car accident can also cause problems; when a seat belt locks to stop your body from being thrown through the windshield, it causes your body to twist as a result of the torque applied by your seatbelt on your shoulder. An airbag deploying will impact your upper body and facial area, which could contribute to pain and damage in your chest, neck, back, and shoulders. If you've ever been in a car or recreational vehicle accident, even a low speed one, you should be aware that there is the potential that the accident caused long-term damage that needs to be examined and corrected.

Sports are another primary concern. As we have gotten more competitive in each sport, physical contact has elevated in almost every circumstance. While the extra activity we experience while playing sports can have big benefits concerning our overall health, collisions experienced during play have the opposite effect. Whether playing around the house, or on a professional team, collisions are bad news for the head and spine.

Nearly everyone is aware of the growing concern regarding concussions, but we don't always think about the impacts on our other body parts. Any collision strong enough to cause a concussion has the potential to cause injury to the spine as well. These injuries happen not just in sports like hockey and football, but nearly all sports. A bad fall on a pair of skates or an awkward trip while running can have as strong an impact as a big hit in a football game. Every fall is different, but each one has the potential to cause misalignment or other injury. You will find more information on concussions at the end of this chapter.

If you have ever moved to a new home or helped a friend relocate their belongings, you've probably done some heavy lifting. When we lift without thinking we often put ourselves in awkward, uncomfortable, and dangerous positions. The human body is remarkable, but lifting heavy objects puts a big strain on our bodies. We can't avoid this type of work all the time, but if we make smart choices we can limit the negative consequences that these actions have on us. Not only smart choices like choosing Chiropractic, but choosing to think about the proper ways to lift an object before actually doing it, and making sure we have enough help so we don't overexert ourselves. Don't forget to warm your muscles up a bit and stretch out before lifting anything heavy!

———————————

I previously mentioned the natural functions of our body. Our spine was created by our body and is maintained by it, but it does have limits. Why can't the body align the spine on its own? To even begin to answer such a question, we need to develop some perspective.

When I was younger, I played basketball often. I had a bad tendency to hurt myself, my fingers in particular. I ended up breaking, dislocating, or jamming nearly all of my fingers at some point during the years I played. What do you do when you or your child dislocates or breaks a bone? Most people go to the doctor to have it set and begin the healing process. Not me. I was stubborn, and I never went. I can tell you from personal experience that the healing process was painful, inefficient, and incomplete. My fingers did heal over time, but they are not like new. Because I didn't take care of them properly when the injury occurred, some of the damage is permanent. They don't move well, they don't bend well, and they certainly aren't straight. My hands and fingers now have very little strength. I wish that I had sought help when I had the chance; I now have to live with the consequences. The idea of having a doctor "set", or realign broken or dislocated bones in your fingers is similar to the general idea of Chiropractic. Chiropractors use several techniques to ensure that your vertebrae are properly aligned. When they are out of place, the chiropractor encourages the bone to move back in to place with a little assistance. If you fracture or break one of your vertebra, unfortunately your chiropractor can't help you much. But they will be happy to do what they can once you've healed, and try to realign your spine.

Your body is unable to do this on its own on a large scale. It can make small changes, but once we have created poor habits or experienced trauma, the body struggles to repair the damage to the spine that we have done. Instead, it will end up making sacrifices in an effort to repair the misalignment. The body may alter the way some muscles are used in an effort to prevent the bones in the spine from shifting even further out of place. In most cases, this is not enough to fix the problem; it is merely enough to prevent the problem from worsening, or delay more permanent damage from occuring. Just as you would visit a regular doctor to have your wrist, shoulder, or finger set back in place, you need to do the same for your back and neck. Your chiropractor is likely very knowledgeable about many of the other joints in the body, and they may be able to align other areas in which you have discomfort, pain, or prior injury.

When you ignore the need for Chiropractic care, you put your entire body at risk. Your spine is the backbone of your body – both literally and figuratively. Any action that negatively impacts your spine is a detriment to your health. The risks of serious injury increase with every poor decision you make; injuries that could include herniated discs, joint degeneration, fused vertebrae, or even paralysis in the most extreme cases. Why does any individual need Chiropractic care? Because the stresses and strains we place on our spine far exceed the limits of its design. Instead of saying, "Why do I need Chiropractic care?" perhaps we should be examining the many ways we put our body in jeopardy every day, and question our reasons for doing so.

Concussions
By Stephanie Foisy Mills, D.C., C.C.W.P.

A concussion is a traumatic injury to the brain that changes the way the brain functions. The obvious mechanism of injury is an impact to the skull. However, concussions can also happen from jolts to the brain caused by a whiplash-type injury. Sports, falls, and motor vehicle accidents account for the majority of concussions. For most people concussion symptoms will clear on their own within ten days, but for others, symptoms such as headaches, dizziness, vision problems, and brain fog can persist for weeks or even months. When symptom duration is longer than two to three weeks, the diagnosis becomes, "Post-Concussion Syndrome." The typical mentality when approaching concussion treatment is to "wait and see," as lingering symptoms will highlight internal damage, dictating future limits and recovery times for patients.

There are no drugs that cure the damage of a concussion. Most drug-based recommendations made by a medical doctor are aimed at quelling the symptoms of the brain injury. For example, attention deficit disorder drugs may be prescribed to help with concentration difficulties, while migraine medication may be used to relieve post-concussion headaches. Neither of these medications help the brain to heal. In fact, they may only be masking the problem and potentially increasing the gravity of the situation. Covering up symptoms could allow a concussed patient to wrongly think he is healed and ready to return to activities, possibly causing further brain injuries or impairing healing. Since a concussion can't be "seen" on an x-ray or traditional MRI, the most common way to assess the progress made by the patient is through an inventory of his or her symptoms. Thus, using medications could skew a patient's self-assessment.

Currently there is no evidence-based standard for treating a concussion. Guidelines such as "Return to Play" have been established by medical experts using the knowledge currently available. More research is needed to understand traumatic brain injuries and how best to help the body heal.

One aspect of concussion management that warrants further investigation is the concurrent presence of vertebral subluxation. There is little doubt that the mechanism of injury (either a forceful head impact or the whipping of the skull and cervical spine) could cause vertebral misalignments. Therefore, we encourage anyone who has a history of concussion to have their spine checked by a chiropractor. Furthermore, for those still suffering from mild traumatic brain injury symptoms, consider looking to your Doctor of Chiropractic as a valuable resource on the road to recovery. Chiropractic adjustments may help with the symptoms of a concussion, and can also help act as a "re-boot" for your brain.

VII.

COMMON PATIENT MISTAKES

By Stephanie Foisy Mills, D.C., C.C.W.P.

Patients want to do the right thing, and they mean well but sometimes they just don't know what they don't know. I have seen and heard some ridiculous things over my years in practice that make me cringe. If only someone had taken us aside in elementary school and taught us the ABC's of spinal health! The fact is, we learned about brushing our teeth, but no one taught us how to take care of our spine and nervous system. We've all made mistakes unknowingly. Please, if you recognize yourself in the following, act now to correct the damage and stop committing these heinous crimes against your spine!

Stomach Sleepers Beware

While catching some nightly zzz's on your stomach may feel comfortable, help you fall asleep, and/or keep you from snoring, it is absolutely an unacceptable way to sleep (unless you can figure out a way to keep your spine neutral while in this position). Most stomach sleeping positions fail to support your lower back, leaving you far more likely to wake up stiff and sore. Worse yet, sleeping belly down may create an unwanted spinal shift and create damage in the neck. Just think about it: most stomach sleepers turn their head to the side to avoid suffocating in the pillow. Many will prefer turning their head to just one side each night. Sleeping every night with your head wrenched and rotated in the same position can cause misalignments of the cervical vertebrae and a loss of the normal forward-shaped curve of the neck.

The ideal position for sleeping is on your back with a small pillow or neck roll to support the normal curve in the neck. You can also place a pillow under your knees for lower back comfort. Sleeping on your side with a pillow of the right thickness for a neutral head is also an approved option. When side sleeping, consider adding a small pillow between your knees and lower legs to maintain hip alignment. While we're on the subject of sleeping, never fall asleep in a recliner or on the couch with your head propped on the arm rest. Ouch!

Smartphone Users Take Caution

Research has been published exposing the risk of a new condition called "text neck", as mentioned in the previous chapter. In my opinion, it is becoming an epidemic. Look around and you will see that people of all ages have their heads dropped downward staring into a screen. It is the forward flexion of the neck that is dangerous.

Medical Doctor Kenneth Hansraj, Chief of Spine Surgery at New York Spine Surgery and Rehabilitation Medicine, examined the increased forces exerted on the neck with poor posture. In his paper published in Surgical Technology International (2014), Dr. Hansraj points out that the human head weighs about a dozen pounds. As the neck bends forward and down, the weight on the cervical spine increases. At a 15-degree angle, the weight of the head is the equivalent of about 27 pounds; at 30 degrees it is 40 pounds; at 60 degrees it is 60 pounds!

Over time, this forward head posture, sometimes referred to as "text neck", can become painful and lead to early wear and tear on the spine. It can even lead to spinal degeneration, or the need for surgery. The earlier text neck is addressed, the better. Your chiropractor can address the structural shifts in your spine that may have already occurred, and now you, as an aware consumer, can change the way you hold your phone while it is in use. My suggestion: bring your phone up in front of your face, rather than bending your head down to it. It is a subtle change that can make a big difference.

Sitting: A Health Hazard

There is the least amount of stress on your spine when it is in a neutral position. Standing puts an average of 100 mm Hg of pressure on the discs of your spine. Sitting, in contrast, increases the intradiscal load to approximately 140 mm Hg. It is even worse if you are a sloucher! The poor posture and structural shifts the body experiences when slouching can cause up to 190mm Hg of pressure on your discs. Poor posture over-stretches spinal ligaments, interrupts blood supply, and can cause aggravated back muscles. The average American sits at least 8 hours per day (most studies agree on this). This increases the risk for spinal misalignments, stress on the discs, and even the possibility of an earlier death.

A study published in the Archives of Internal Medicine (Banks, Bauman, Chey, Korda, & van der Ploeg, 2012) found that those who sat for more than eight hours a day had a 15 percent greater risk of dying within three years than those who sat for fewer than four hours a day. Those who sat for 11 hours or more a day had a 40 percent greater risk of early death. What may be surprising is that this risk still held true for those who regularly dedicated time to exercise. Since it seems that you can't exercise away the negative effects of sitting, the obvious solution is: sit less! Developments in workplace ergonomics have made standing work stations more readily available and cost effective. I encourage you to check out the standing desk options to create an office where you can think and work on your feet.

If you've got a desk job and are not ready to move to a standing work station, then I have a few other suggestions for you. First, consider using a large Yoga/Pilates ball instead of a chair. The ball requires your trunk muscles to fire to keep you balanced. There is more opportunity for micro-movements which encourage fluid exchange in your joints.

If you are using a traditional chair, place a lumbar

roll between your lower back and your chair. You can purchase a lumbar support, or just use a bath towel rolled to the size of your forearm. You can use this when driving, as well. When sitting in a chair, keep your feet flat on the floor. Don't cross one leg underneath you, or sit on one of your feet. Likewise, don't cross your legs at the ankle. If you are using a computer monitor it should be positioned straight ahead of you, so that the top of the monitor is at least at eye level.

Ideally you should sit or stand so that your eyes are about 2-3 inches below the top of the monitor. If you have a laptop it is virtually impossible to have good ergonomics. Your keyboard should be low, at arm level, but the monitor needs to be high to assure for a neutrally positioned cervical spine. A low screen causes you to look down, flexing the cervical spine and putting added pressure on the cervical discs as noted above. If you utilize a laptop, consider investing in a separate keyboard so you can move your screen to a safer height, or purchase a secondary screen for home use.

Self-Cracking, Popping, and Home-Manipulation

Please, do not try to crack your own back. It may be a habit, and it may even appear to give you temporary "relief" from pain or tightness, but in actuality it may be worsening your condition. Popping your own neck or back (or having a friend walk on your back) is not the same as having a Doctor of Chiropractic carefully assess your spine, determine which vertebrae to move and in what direction, and how much force to use. Home manipulation can be downright dangerous.

If you've already fallen into this nasty trap, it's a sign that you intuitively know that there is a problem in your spine. But let me assure you, you'll never be able to truly fix it yourself. Even chiropractors can't adjust themselves. So please, just say, "no" to self-cracking, and leave it to the professionals.

Efficacy of Chiropractic Adjustments versus Self-Manipulation of the Lumbar Spine in a 17-year-old Male with Chronic Low Back Pain: A Case Study

This study documents a patient who began habitually self-manipulating his lower back after he suffered an injury weight lifting. His low back pain worsened over the period of a year, until he sought Chiropractic care. His Chiropractic examination revealed areas of hypermobility (too much movement) and also areas of segmental hypomobility (too little movement - think "stuck" vertebrae).

Pain medications and injections by his medical provider proved ineffective. The authors identify that in order to provide lower back pain relief, specific Chiropractic adjustments were performed three times per week for a period of three months. The study's authors concluded that "this case suggests that specific high-velocity low-amplitude Chiropractic adjustments are safer and more effective at treating low back pain than self-manipulating, and that non-specific self-manipulation can exacerbate current problems in patients."

(Windwer & Wolfman, 2015, p. 46)

Wardrobe Woes

The single biggest offender for men in regards to their wardrobe is their wallets. It is not the wallet that is the problem, it is the location. Never, ever put your wallet in your back pocket and then sit on it. Not only can it compress the piriformis muscle and irritate the sciatic nerve, but it can also result in a bad shift in your pelvis. Sitting on a wallet (especially a loaded one) raises the hip corresponding to the side the wallet is located on. Most men I have met carry their wallet on the same side day after day. Your pelvis serves as the foundation to your spine. If it becomes misaligned, then the rest of your spine above will shift, subluxate, and compensate for the issues at the bottom. It is best to carry your wallet in your front pocket, or be diligent about removing it when you sit in your car, at your desk, or any other place.

Women: as a vertically challenged female, I can appreciate the height gained by wearing high heels. I also love the many colors, styles, and brands I can collect to create the perfect look. Our legs may look better in heels, but our spines and feet pay the price. If there is one piece of women's fashion most responsible for causing spinal subluxations, pelvic shifts, and other structural issues, it is definitely high heels.

Instead of distributing weight over the entire foot and utilizing the three normal arches, being in a heel flattens the transverse arch and forces weight onto the metatarsal bones at their heads. Over time the loss of the medial longitudinal arch causes the head of the first metatarsal to deviate medially and can result in unsightly and painful bunions. Wearing heels (even small ones) causes the pelvis to shift, putting stress on the sacroiliac joints and the lumbosacral junction. I won't say never wear them, because that is unrealistic to most of us. But please, limit them to special occasions, not daily ritual.

Bags and carry-all's are necessary accessories but please use caution. If you carry a laptop, a back-pack-style bag, with weight distributed equally over both shoulders, is far more advantageous to your spine than a single strap over the shoulder or an across-the-body design. When shopping for a backpack for yourself or your child, look for one with wide, padded straps. It is great to purchase a backpack with a waist and/or chest strap to disperse the weight to your torso. Some backpacks even come with lumbar support. Experts say that children should never carry a backpack weighing more than 10-15% of their body weight, but the exact numbers vary with each source consulted. For active adults, especially long distance hikers, the best advice I can give is to make sure that you are not over packing! The lighter the better.

Starting Baby off Right

How you handle your children, from the very moment they are born, impacts their spinal health. While we will be discussing pediatric Chiropractic care in a later chapter, allow me to address a few parenting habits here. If you are not a chiropractor, you have probably never given much thought to some of these things.

63

For example, when changing diapers, don't grab only one leg – instead lift both legs together. Do not twist the baby's pelvis or lower back, keep both legs at the same height off the changing table. Likewise, be careful not to lift the baby's legs too high, which could put stress or strain on his neck. If you're using disposable diapers, never press the tape down against baby's hip, instead do it against your index finger. Also, be sure to give your baby sufficient tummy time to allow for development of trunk musculature, back extensors, and shoulder girdle muscles.

Avoid using jumpers, baby walkers, and exersaucers! The biggest problem with these items are that they place baby's spine in a load-bearing position before the spine is developmentally ready to do so. Walkers also prevent children from seeing their feet, grabbing things, and exploring/investigating their environment. And of course, make it a routine to have your baby's spine checked after birth and regularly throughout their first year of life by your family chiropractor.

References

Banks, E., Bauman, A., Chey, T., Korda, R. J., & van der Ploeg, H. P. (2012). Sitting time and all-cause mortality risk in 222,297 Australian adults. Archives of Internal Medicine, 494-500. doi:10.1001/archinternmed.2011.2174

Hansraj, K. K. (2014). Assessment of stresses in the cervical spine caused by posture and position of the head. Surgical Technology International(XXV), 277-279.

Windwer, S., & Wolfman, M. (2015, April). Efficacy of Chiropractic adjustments versus self-manipulation of the lumbar spine in a 17-year-old male with chronic low back pain: A case study. Annals of Vertebral Subluxation Research, 43-47.

Additional Resources

Chiropractic Works: Adjusting to a Higher Quality of Life by Timothy J. Feuling

VIII.
SPECIAL CASES

By Justin C. Chase and Stephanie Foisy Mills, D.C., C.C.W.P.

Caring for Youth

When entities are in their infancy, they are at their most delicate. This is as true for a child as it is for a plant, an animal, or even a business. A newborn child faces many challenges. Their bodies have not fully developed and many aspects of their skeletal structure remain too weak to adequately protect them in all situations. An accident can lead to damage in the structure and health of our young, and that damage may persist throughout their lives.

In addition to physical concerns, the brain continues developing well into our twenties, and our body is constantly adding to or reworking the system of neurons that reach throughout it. This system extends, as we recall from previous chapters, down the spinal cord as part of the central nervous system, and then to the extremities of the body to make up the peripheral nervous system. Because these neural connections are so crucial to most functions of our body, it is clear that spinal health is a concern for all of us – but newborns, infants, and adolescents may be even more susceptible to the harm that could result from the presence of subluxations.

Chiropractors are trained in very gentle techniques for adjusting infants, and use different evaluation methods designed specifically for children whose bodies are still developing.

There is evidence that suggests that adjusting an infant can lead to the resolution of certain problems. Misaligned vertebrae in infants are associated with problems like colic, difficulty latching or breastfeeding, and even problems with bowel elimination. A study conducted by the National Health Service and a private clinic in Copenhagen, Denmark (Nilsson, Nordsteen, & Wiberg, 1999) examined two groups of infants, recording daily hours of crying in a colic diary. One group was treated with the drug dimethicone (used in diaper cream to prevent rash and irritation) for two weeks in an effort to reduce colic, while the other group received Chiropractic adjustments for the same length of time.

The study demonstrated that Chiropractic adjustments reduced crying time by more than twice that of the use of dimethicone. With no medication or other alterations in the children's lifestyles, Chiropractic reduced crying time by well over two hours per day for infants! It certainly appears that there is a correlation between Chiropractic and the comfort of a young child. Further research is necessary to determine exactly how correcting subluxations impacts the length of time spent crying by infants.

Issues like chronic ear infections, attention deficits, constipation, asthma, or other symptoms may be associated with vertebral subluxations in children. Subluxations affect the nervous system and the ability of an individual to interpret and interact with their environment. In a case study by Lathrop and Yoshimura on a five-year-old girl published in the Annals of Vertebral Subluxation Research (2015), the effect of Chiropractic adjustment was examined with regards to the child's sensory processing disorder, difficulty sleeping, developmental delays, and other functional disorders. After receiving adjustments via the Activator Technique, objective indicators showed that the patient had improved functioning in bowel elimination, mood, ability to concentrate, and experienced more restful sleep.

Supporting the proper structure and function of the body at a young age can lead to fewer problems down the road as our children begin to engage in activities like walking, running, and playing sports. The results of these everyday activities can lead to spinal shifts that alter the structural integrity of the spine. Since children's spines are still developing, early misalignments can lead to irreversible damage. It makes sense, then, that properly maintaining and aligning the spine in a growing child can lead to a healthier, more resilient spine as an adult – which in turn leads to a healthier adult life.

Maternity Care

Over the span of nine months, pregnant women's bodies go through dramatic changes. One of those changes includes carrying an additional 25-35 pounds of weight in the midsection, which can naturally result in back pain. In a published paper, 75% of pregnant women reported that they experienced relief from pain while under Chiropractic care (Shaw, 2003). Let's take a basic look at the unique structural issues of pregnancy to understand why.

The normal weight gain along with a growing baby can increase stress on the sacro-iliac (SI) joints. The weight of the baby also causes the pelvis to tip forward, anteriorly, and reduces the normal lordosis (forward curve) of the lower back. Both can result in back pain or sciatica, which is when pain travels from the low back or buttocks down the leg, towards the calf and/or foot. Further, increased breast tissue weight can put stress on mom's mid-back, causing mid-back and neck pain. As her center of gravity changes and postural shifts occur, mom's head may translate forward, causing an extension of the head on the first vertebra. This could easily result in neck pain and/or headaches.

Chiropractic adjustments to reduce spinal misalignments are a welcome pain reliever for moms-to-be. With less pain women are able to stay active and continue to exercise throughout their pregnancy, which further improves their health and birth experience. But the value in Chiropractic care during pregnancy is much richer than "just" feeling better and staying active.

It makes sense that regular attention to the pelvis, spine, soft tissues and nervous system function throughout pregnancy would make labor more efficient. Researcher Joan Fallon, D.C., investigated the impact of Chiropractic adjustments on labor times (Fallon, 1994, p. 52, 109). She found that first-time mothers receiving Chiropractic care during pregnancy experienced a 24% reduction in labor time compared to average, while those giving birth for the second or third time had an impressive 39% reduction in labor time.

Chiropractic care helps to normalize alignment and function of the pelvis and can reduce musculoskeletal causes of intra-uterine constraint, which can promote proper presentation of the baby during delivery. While the goal of Chiropractic care is not to turn a breech baby, many babies have improved their positioning from breech to a head-down presentation following Chiropractic care that addressed mom's pelvic subluxations. Chiropractic care, especially when utilizing the Webster Technique, can improve pelvic balance and make more room for the baby to grow comfortably (Pistolese, 2002).

It is also plausible to conclude that adjustments for pregnant moms could be beneficial to outcomes of delivery by looking at osteopathic research. In a retrospective study, researchers examined medical records of 160 women from four cities who received prenatal osteopathic manipulation, comparing them to 161 randomly selected records of women from the same cities (Arsenault, et al., 2003). The second group of women were selected from among those who did not receive prenatal osteopathic manipulations. The researchers found a significantly associated reduction of meconium-stained amniotic fluid and preterm delivery and a marginally significant reduction in the use of forceps for the group that had received prenatal osteopathic manipulations.

Lastly, for those cautious or concerned, Chiropractic care for the pregnant woman has been given for over one hundred years and is considered safe. There are many places, such as the American Pregnancy Association, that recommend Chiropractic for pregnant women, acknowledging that chiropractors are trained to treat patients who are pregnant.

Senior Care

Many Americans over the age of sixty-five take multiple prescriptions daily. Some of these medications are intended to counteract the results of aging as the body begins to break down, but some are prescribed solely to reduce pain. Even if seniors who came in for Chiropractic care were only able to reduce their need for pain medications, this would be a huge benefit to them.

Chiropractors are able to help individuals overcome many of the aches and pains in joints throughout the body by ensuring they are properly aligned and that bones are in their correct positions, which allows for further range of motion. This in turn can lead to increased comfort in everyday activities, making it more plausible for seniors to stay active, fit, and able to care for themselves effectively. Most seniors that I know would prefer to remain independent and be responsible for themselves – and when they can do this, they often lead happier, healthier lives.

Since Chiropractic has shown promise in leading to improved body functions over time (including digestion, elimination, breathing, and blood pressure, among others), it would follow that Chiropractic would be beneficial for seniors. Although seniors have much higher risk of injury in general, the risks associated with senior Chiropractic care remain minimal. A good chiropractor will perform a thorough examination and look at the complete patient history in order to determine if it is necessary to employ a gentler adjusting technique. As with any patient, adjustments will be made relative to the condition of the spine and any existing subluxations, ensuring that the treatment is appropriate and beneficial for the patient.

Although the ideal situation would be that everyone received Chiropractic care from the time they were born until the time they moved on, this is unrealistic in many cases. Though it may be too late to undo some of the damage a lifetime of disregard for the spine can cause, it is never too late to make improvements. Even when complete correction of long-term spinal shifts is unrealistic, seniors can still benefit greatly from receiving Chiropractic care. At the bare minimum, beginning care as a senior can help to prevent further degeneration of the spine due to the presence of subluxations.

In addition to the bodily benefits that seniors may see from Chiropractic care, there are studies that indicate that seniors receiving Chiropractic adjustments can save a significant amount of money. One such study by Manello, Rupert, and Sandefur examined 311 Chiropractic patients receiving maintenance or wellness care for five years or longer (2000). These patients spent only 31% of the national average for health care services for people in this age range. The patients receiving Chiropractic care also visited a medical provider 50% fewer times than their comparable peers. This means that on average, for every thousand dollars a 'regular' senior spends on medical care, a senior who has been receiving Chiropractic adjustments for five years or longer will typically spend only three hundred ten dollars.

It is clear that Chiropractic offers significant benefits for seniors, regardless of their current physical condition. There is also the benefit of visiting a clinic with a supportive staff that can help keep seniors aware of new health information, encourage them to be active, and help them eat in ways that can promote their longevity. There is a place in Chiropractic for everyone, and seniors are no exception. It is never too late to begin making positive changes in your life, and Chiropractic often leads to many positive outcomes.

References

Arsenault, D., Johnson, K., King, H., Lockwood, M., Quist, R., & Tettambel, M. (2003, December). Ostepathic manipulative treatment in prenatal care: A retrospective case control design study. Journal of the American Osteopathic Association, 103, 577-582.

Fallon, J. M. (1994). Textbook on Chiropractic & pregnancy. Arlington, Virginia: International Chiropractic Association.

Lathrop, J. M., & Yoshimura, R. (2015, May). Improvement in sensory modulation & functional disorders in a female pediatric patient undergoing Chiropractic care. Annals of Vertebral Subluxation Research, 108-118.

Manello, D., Rupert, R. L., & Sandefur, R. (2000). Maintenance care: Health promotion services administered to US Chiropractic patients ages 65 and older, part II. Journal of Manipulative and Physiological Therapeutics, 23(1), 10-19.

Nilsson, N., Nordsteen, J., & Wiberg, J. (1999, October)

The short-term effect of spinal manipulation in the treatment of Infantile Colic: A randomized controlled clinical trial with a blinded observer. Journal of Manipulative Physiological Therapeutics, 517-522.

Pistolese, R. A. (2002). The Webster technique: a Chiropractic technique with obstetric implications. Journal of Manipulative Physiological Therapeutics, E1-E9.

Shaw, G. (2003). When to adjust: Chiropractic and pregnancy. Journal of American Chiropractic Association, 8-16.

Additional Resources

Holistic Moms Network
http://www.holisticmoms.org/
International Chiropractic Pediatric Association
http://www.icpa4kids.org/

IX.
WELLNESS CARE

By Stephanie Foisy Mills, D.C., C.C.W.P.

One of the biggest myths and misconceptions around Chiropractic care is that once you start going, you'll always have to go. On one hand, this couldn't be farther from the truth; as a member of a free society you have a choice (for the most part) about what you do with your body. But on the other hand, once you've established a positive habit and are reaping the benefits, it doesn't make sense to stop. Therefore, many Chiropractic patients end up *choosing* to make Chiropractic care a part of their health strategy – for life.

This analogy may gross you out, but will necessarily illustrate why patients continue returning for Chiropractic care. Imagine your parents never taught you to brush your teeth. There was not a single toothbrush in your home. By first grade, no doubt, your mouth would be foul smelling and your teeth would be yellow, fuzzy and downright disgusting. That would be "normal" for you. You simply wouldn't know any different. Your oral hygiene takes a turn though, after an angel from dental heaven pays a visit to your elementary classroom. She teaches you why to brush, the approved brushing technique, and even presents you with your own toothbrush, toothpaste, and floss. She then performs a cleaning of your teeth so that you leave school with a fresh, minty mouth full of smooth, glossy, and clean teeth for the first time in your life. You love the feel of it; you're proud to smile, and your friends are thankful too. Wouldn't you choose to brush again the next day? After learning what you'd been missing out on, it now makes more sense to adopt this habit and continue it for life.

Chiropractic "maintenance" or "wellness" care is similar. It is a choice that makes sense. It is continuing an activity that makes you feel better, improves your appearance and posture, and helps your body function at a higher level. Ongoing maintenance care is a natural extension of your intensive corrective care. The duration of the corrective phase varies, but your chiropractor will know when the time is appropriate to move you towards a maintenance phase. She will reduce the frequency of your spinal check-ups based on your progress, as demonstrated by improvements since your initial Chiropractic findings. This could be any combination of thermography improvements, postural changes, palpation exam changes, and/or improved structure as evidenced by re-evaluation x-rays.

Your chiropractor may recommend wellness care as weekly office visits, every other week, or even routine monthly check-ups. Typically these proceed on a schedule, with interval re-evaluations as the practitioner sees fit. However, there are instances where you may want to consider increasing the frequency of your schedule: when you're feeling under the weather, if you're under increased amounts of stress in your life, or if you've physically exerted yourself beyond your capabilities (by shoveling, doing yard work, moving furniture, etc.). Your chiropractor may also recommend a re-evaluation or change in frequency if you begin to experience body signals (symptoms) or if you've experienced a new physical trauma like a fall or car accident.

There are things you can do at home to improve the ability of your body to "hold" wellness adjustments. Incorporate a stretching and spinal hygiene routine into your day. Include both aerobic and anaerobic exercise along with weight lifting into your fitness regimen. Make an effort to follow your chiropractor's nutritional recommendations. As we learned in Healthy Lifestyles, the foods we choose to fuel our bodies with are the substrates for building new cells. The old saying, "Garbage in, garbage out," applies perfectly here. Minimize the damage and maximize the healing by eating whole fresh foods, and by focusing on consuming organic fruits and vegetables as part of a hunter-gatherer diet. And perhaps most importantly, keep your mental fitness in check as well. In other words, control your stress! The following studies highlight the value of wellness care.

Chiropractic Health and Savings Potential

In a study looking back 7 years on over 70,000 "member-months", Cambron, Sarnat, and Winterstein examined differences in medical attention and spending by patients whose primary care providers were doctors of Chiropractic against those who had a doctor of conventional medicine as a PCP. The patients with PCP's who were chiropractors saw noticeably lower rates of medical need, showing decreases of 62% in outpatient surgery, a 60.2% reduction of in-hospital admissions, and a 59% decrease in days spent in the hospital. They also experienced a significant decrease of 85% in pharmaceutical costs compared with the patients whose PCP's were conventional doctors.

(Cambron, Sarnat, & Winterstein, 2007)

Athletic Ability

Chiropractic care improves quality of life and overall body performance. Professional athletes and sports teams know this and have included doctors of Chiropractic on their healthcare teams for years. One study compared 24 asymptomatic athletes, measured at six and twelve weeks of care and compared them to 22 control athletes in terms of speed, agility, balance and power. The researchers found greater improvements in the group receiving Chiropractic care and concluded that correcting the subluxation complex helps the body perform at a higher level. In a specific activity measuring reaction speeds of the hand in response to a visual stimulus, the control group only improved by 1% over 6 weeks, while the group receiving adjustments improved by 18%, eventually improving by 30% over the full 12 weeks.

(Lauro & Mouch, 1991)

References

Cambron, J. A., Sarnat, R. L., & Winterstein, J. (2007, May). Clinical utilization and cost outcomes from an integrative medicine independent physician association: An additional three year update. Journal of Manipulative and Physiological Therapeutics, 30(4), 263-269.

Lauro, A., & Mouch, B. (1991). Chiropractic effects on athletic ability. The Journal of Chiropractic Research and Clinical Investigation, 84-87.

X.

THE CHIROPRACTIC "MIRACLE"

By Justin C. Chase

There are many different definitions of the word, "miracle." This word is defined with religious and spiritual overtones and with a sense of awe in relation to the unknown. While it has proven impossible to identify a single, consistent definition of what a miracle truly consists of, let us define it here as:

> **Miracle:** *An event or situation with a favorable result that is highly unexpected and inexplicable with our present levels of knowledge.*

What is considered a miracle in one part of the world may be taken as an everyday occurrence in another part. Notable events of the past were likely considered miracles, yet we may take them for granted today because of the knowledge we gained in trying to understand them.

When we lack sufficient knowledge to offer up a satisfactory explanation for an event that has occurred, we look at it with a sense of wonder and awe. But the doctors and scientists among us move beyond those emotions, searching for a cause and seeking to understand how events unfolded as they did. They seek not only to understand why these things happened, but how they happened, so that they can be studied and repeated. In this way, we make progress as a society and unlock new knowledge, providing us access to things that we previously had only dreamt about.

Until recently (the past few centuries), humans had little knowledge of the ways that certain chemicals affected the body. We knew that certain plants and compounds would have an effect on the body, but we didn't know how these things worked. The truth is, we still don't have a complete understanding. Although we now have a much stronger picture of how our bodies will react to certain chemicals, we still can't explain everything that transpires as a result of their introduction into the body.

While some things are predictable, we still have a limited knowledge of the human body and we cannot account for the immense number of complexities it contains. This is evidenced in the medicines, treatments, and surgeries we use today – they still result in some very unpredictable outcomes, debilitating side effects, and sometimes even permanent damage. New drugs often cure diseases of one type, but facilitate several others. This is not unique to drugs that fight life-threatening conditions; nearly every drug we use has some side effects because we cannot account for all of the variables within the human body.

If we look at the number of people in the world who

are relatively healthy, we can see that the human body does a remarkable job on its own. Despite the artificial foods we ingest, the reduction in our physical lifestyles, and the intake of chemicals with every breath we take, our bodies have managed to survive on their own. We have made improvements in our medical care, but often these improvements have been dictated by the damages we have inflicted upon ourselves. Look at the people you know who most actively reflect what human life is meant to be – look at those who eat natural foods, who are active day in and day out, those who think and live with purpose – I think you will find that they are often the healthiest among us.

We may consider it a miracle today when someone lives a long, healthy life. This would represent a contradiction of our definition of a miracle, for two reasons. First, it will be a sad day when we say that our expectation of a newborn child is that they will *not* live a long and healthy life. I certainly hope that, barring a disability or birth defect, this isn't the expectation we have for a newborn. Second, there is an explanation for a human who lives a long and healthy life, which means it is not a miracle. The explanation is that they are living as they are meant to, that they have been allowed to grow and thrive as they needed, and that they have maintained the structure that is necessary to protect their body. We don't have to understand every intricacy of the human body to know that it works.

What we *should* consider a miracle is the human body itself. It is versatile, adaptable, and incredibly complex. Just when we think we know how it works or what it is capable of, we find something unexpected. Although

82

we understand many aspects of how it works, we are nowhere near understanding it in full. It fits our definition of a miracle perfectly. When we look at all the things our bodies are capable of, it is difficult not to be in awe. What, though, does Chiropractic have to do with miracles?

Chiropractic has been associated with many miracle cases over time. When we think of these miracles, we often gravitate towards the most extreme examples. There have been case studies (though few officially documented) of chiropractors adjusting patients who have been in comas – patients who then recovered shortly after these adjustments, despite having been in the coma for weeks or months. There are also other, less extreme events that leave us wanting an explanation. Four of these cases are summarized as follows:

Resolution of Multiple Syptoms

There is the case of a nine-year old, who had been delivered with the use of forceps, suffering from Tourettes Syndrome, ADHD, depression, asthma, insomnia, and headaches. This child was on several medications, and was being monitored by a doctor as well as by his parents. After an initial examination, a cervical subluxation was identified and treatment began. After six weeks of care, it was identified by his practicing doctor, both parents, and the patient's own description that all of his symptoms had disappeared. He was taken off of all but one small dose of medicine, and after five months all symptoms remained nonexistent.

(Elster, Upper Cervical Chiropractic Care For A Nine-Year-Old Male With Tourette Syndrome, Attention Deficit Hyperactivity Disorder, Depression, Asthma, Insomnia, and Headaches: A Case Report, 2003)

Improved Nursing Habits

A two-day old newborn was showing problems nursing and was unable to latch. The baby also showed signs of lethargy and a yellowish tinge to her skin color. Considered hypothyroid by a medical doctor, the baby was recommended to be hospitalized, but received a Chiropractic adjustment to correct a left lateral listing of her head. Immediately after, the baby began to nurse on her own and the other symptoms cleared in time.

(Esch, 1988)

Overcoming Tension Headaches

Another case involved a thirty-five year old woman with daily migraine and tension headaches who had sustained a concussion at the age of twenty-three. She had been a professional ice skater, and had reported no other health problems prior to the accident. After the concussion the migraines and tension headaches appeared, and despite taking medications these problems persisted for twelve years. After an upper cervical subluxation was identified and corrected, all headaches became absent three months into care. Her case was monitored and evaluated by a doctor, the patient's subjective descriptions, and the use of thermographic scans. After one year, her chronic migraines and tension headaches were still gone.

(Elster, Upper Cervical Chiropractic Care for a Patient with Chronic Migraine Headaches with an Appendix Summarizing an Additional 100 Headache Cases, 2003)

X. THE CHIROPRACTIC "MIRACLE"

Facilitating Motor Skills

A child with a transient motor tic, exhibiting shoulder shrugging, eye rolling every 3-5 seconds, and arching of the neck and back with an open mouth was found to have several subluxations. The atlas, C7, T4, and sacroiliac joint were adjusted six times over a five week period, after which the motor tic disorder and other symptoms cleared. Following an ice-skating fall, eye blinking and rolling reappeared, and the patient returned for additional care. This was about two-and-a-half months after the initial care. Once again, following Chiropractic adjustments, symptoms cleared.

(Alcantara, Davis, & Oman, 2009)

Each of these miracles indicates the ability of the body to heal itself given some needed assistance, *not* the ability of Chiropractic to create miracles. Doctors of Chiropractic are well aware of how to facilitate the correction of subluxations and how to maintain the natural structure of the body.

What no one can predict is precisely what changes the body makes in response to Chiropractic care. Chiropractic is a tool used by doctors to assist the body in performing its natural functions in order to allow it to operate at peak efficiency. The miracles we see are not the result of Chiropractic, they are the result of the body healing itself. This is one of the foundations that Chiropractic is based upon.

It has been said that Chiropractic care can result in significant changes in the body, often different for each individual. Some find the relief of pain, increased flexibility, or a boundless sense of energy. Others find relief from migraines, mental disorders, or concussion symptoms. Still others find they are able to have a baby following Chiropractic care despite years of failed fertility treatments. People find they have fewer allergies, an easier time going to the bathroom, increased eyesight, a reduction of seizures, improvement in diabetes, reduced blood pressure, resolution of insomnia – the list goes on and on.

Thinking that Chiropractic is the cause of all these changes makes very little sense. Think about it. Though doctors use a variety of different techniques, many different changes will be seen in patients with the same doctor. To think that the same type of treatment is the cause of all these different and miraculous results is illogical. Would you expect a doctor treating your broken leg to somehow stop your runny nose, or fix your poor eyesight?

Doctors of Chiropractic work to improve the structure and the function of the spine, as well as other joints in the body. They let your body do the rest. They realize that the miracle is not in the science or art that they practice, but in the philosophy behind it – the philosophy that the body possesses an innate intelligence, and can heal itself if its proper form and function are maintained. The miracle is within you.

———————

There are those who say that Chiropractic is a fraud, because there is no proof that it leads to the changes people associate it with. This is irrational, and nonsensical. First, Chiropractic has proof that the techniques used by doctors work. Their purpose is to realign the spine and care for the numerous joints throughout the body. The techniques used are tried and true. When properly administered, they fulfill that purpose. This is all the proof needed to show that Chiropractic works. What follows from these changes is beyond the scope of Chiropractic. The human body is not controlled by any doctor.

There is ongoing research about what connection the manipulations chiropractors perform have with the rest of the human body. It is likely that eventually we will know enough to assist the body in more exacting ways in an effort to solve specific problems. A portion of the profits from this book will be donated to the Foundation for Vertebral Subluxation, which has ongoing research, scholarship, education, and policy programs in existence for the further understanding of Chiropractic. Chiropractic may never be the cause of the miracles we see it correlated to, but studying the effects of adjustments over time may help us better understand the miracle that is the human body.

What is the "Chiropractic Miracle?" It is the human body's ability to heal itself in ways that we can't even begin to understand yet. It is the incredible complexity that is the human body, which can perform amazing feats when we take care of it properly. Chiropractic may not cause miracles, but it is quite clear that it helps to facilitate them.

References

Alcantara, J., Davis, A., & Oman, R. E. (2009). The effects of Chiropractic on a child with transient motor tics using Gonstead & Toggle techniques. Journal of Pediatric, Maternal & Family Health - Chiropractic(2), 1-9.

Elster, E. (2003). Upper cervical Chiropractic care for a nine-year-old male with Tourette Syndrome, Attention Deficit Hyperactivity Disorder, Depression, Asthma, Insomnia, and headaches: A case report. Journal of Vertebral Subluxation Research, 1-11.

Elster, E. (2003). Upper cervical Chiropractic care for a patient with chronic migraine headaches with an appendix summarizing an additional 100 headache cases. Journal of Vertebral Subluxation Research, 1-10.

Esch, S. (1988). Newborn with atlas subluxation/absent rooting reflex from case reports in Chiropractic pediatrics. ACA Journal of Chiropractic.

Additional Resources

Foundation for Vertebral Subluxation Research
http://www.vertebralsubluxation.org/

Our Daily Meds: How the Pharmaceutical Companies Transformed Themselves into Slick Marketing Machines and Hooked the Nation on Prescription Drugs by Melody Petersen

Overdosed America: The Broken Promise of American Medicine by John Abramson

XI.

DECISION TIME

By Justin C. Chase

At this point, you face a challenge – a crossroads of sorts. You should have a good idea of what Chiropractic is, and why you need it. In the Appendix, you will find information on how you can obtain care – or better yet, you may already have visited a chiropractor. In either case, you should be more informed about eating healthy, exercising, and making smart choices to care for your body. The question is, "What are you going to do about it?"

It is relatively easy to spend a few minutes a day learning about how to care for your body, but it is another thing entirely to begin acting upon that knowledge. As we have suggested throughout this book, starting small and making incremental changes is usually the best approach. Dr. Stephanie mentioned earlier that when it comes to the diet, sometimes the best thing we can do is to begin by adding healthy foods to our meal, eating those first. By doing so we will often feel full sooner and refrain from eating the poor foods we had intended to eat. Over time, we will choose smaller portions of unhealthy food and grow to enjoy the healthy pieces in our diet as we become more used to them. We, of course, should be paying attention to the number of calories we consume in addition to our other dietary changes. Too high of an intake will lead to weight gain, and we all know that in most cases this leads to further health problems.

When we consider how to incorporate exercise regimens into our lives, the easiest way may be to join a gym. It provides easy access to machines and equipment, and sometimes offers a bit of support from employees or people you may meet there. It can, however, get lonely. For people who are not historically successful going to the gym, finding a community to exercise with can be much more effective. See if there are jogging groups near you, obstacle course training sessions, or even just a group of friends who go walking together. Social media allows us to find these types of events at local parks, gyms, and businesses. Sometimes even schools will have programs for kids and adults to exercise!

If you can't find a group, start one with co-workers, friends, or family. Information on beginner exercise activities and long-term planning is easy to find on the internet or in health and fitness books. In the end, so long as you make a change and continue improving upon it, you will see positive results.

The key to making smart choices is to think. Be conscious of the way that you are living your life. It is easy for most people to turn a blind eye, acting as if the failure to acknowledge something means that it doesn't exist. Ignoring our poor choices only hurts us. Start looking at everything that you do, and determine if you could do it better. Think about your posture, the way you move, how you perform your job, and how you drive in your car. The most effective changes for our body may be those that relate to our repeated activities, because a poor decision gets performed over and over again. If you constantly try to make small improvements by actively thinking and finding solutions for the problems you identify, I think you will be amazed at the changes that will result over time.

I hope that you have spent some serious time thinking about the goals you were encouraged to begin identifying earlier in the book. These goals are what will make the changes you implement sustainable - knowing what these changes will do for you in regards to how you want to live your life, and what you will be able to accomplish. This book has been about much more than Chiropractic, it has been about you. In essence, though, that is also what Chiropractic is all about. We wanted you to come to your own conclusions regarding Chiropractic.

I mentioned that you are at a crossroads. The decision you make has the potential to change the way you live. We have established that there is very minimal risk in receiving Chiropractic care, much less than going in for surgery or taking medication full of warnings about side effects. They say that with no risk there can be no reward - but when it comes to your body, how much risk is acceptable? Here, there is minimal risk and the potential for great reward.

It is up to you what you wish to do. I cannot force you to seek care, nor would I even if I could. I will not even tell you to do it. What I would love for you to do is to think about it. Think long and hard about what your life means to you, and what you would do to preserve it, prolong it, or improve it. I think you would be willing to do a lot more than seek out a chiropractor. The effort required to improve your life is minimal compared to the efforts you take every day to live it. So I ask you, in closing, a very simple question that I doubt you will be able to find a sufficient answer for: "Why *wouldn't* you seek Chiropractic care?"

Appendix A:
Where to Start?

By Justin C. Chase

Before you make the decision to set foot inside a Chiropractic office, there are things you can do on your own to start taking better care of your life. The first step is identifying the aspects that are contributing to poor behavior. We'll talk more about making smart choices later; for now the best thing to do is identify the routines and habits in your life that are most detrimental to your body. Making a few small changes now, before visiting a chiropractor, can help your body become more responsive to care, and make you more likely to accomplish the goals you have set for yourself.

Nearly every lifestyle book on the market mentions exercise, nutrition, and sleep as the primary elements of a healthy life. It follows, then, that these should be receiving some level of attention on a daily basis. Making large-scale, drastic changes in your diet is extremely difficult to maintain, so I would suggest starting small.

If you haven't read a nutrition book, start there. Each source is going to have its own perspectives on what constitutes a "healthy" diet, but they'll have consistencies overall. Most of us have a good idea of what we shouldn't be eating. Many chiropractors will refer you to a Paleo-style diet, so be sure to include one of those in your readings.

When trying to make these small dietary changes, think about cutting processed foods, particularly those high in sugar and saturated fat. Snack foods, candy, and fried foods are all things you can eat less frequently. Adding fruits and vegetables to the diet is certainly going to help - mix up your food intakes and eat all different kinds. If you focus on replacing foods you know are bad for you with ones that are better, the changes will be much easier to stick to, and you can continue to improve on them over time. Dr. Stephanie also mentioned in her Healthy Lifestyles chapter that you can start with adding one healthy item to each meal, and then gradually start removing some of the less healthy portions.

It would also be very beneficial for you to monitor and log your diet. Again, there are many apps and programs that can be used. Try to choose one that monitors not only calories, but also nutrients like vitamins and minerals. After a few weeks of monitoring, you can compare your diet with the recommendations for a healthy diet based on your age, height, and weight. You can use the results to determine what foods you need to add or remove from your diet. Many of the programs used to track your diet are included with the purchase of a fitness tracker.

Be aware that most of these programs will likely have high recommendations for grain-related foods, often based on the USDA's food recommendations. Do yourself a favor, though - do a little research on grains and you will probably see that they have little nutritional value: specifically, that they do not contain anything that can't be found in other foods. As far as carbohydrates are concerned, fruits and vegetables are significantly more nutrient dense than grains (much greater nutritional value per calorie). With few nutrients to add to the diet, grains end up contributing excess calories, leaving unused glucose floating in the bloodstream that ends up being converted to fat.

The technological advances over the last decade have allowed us to become more aware of our physical activity than ever. With dozens of fitness trackers in all price ranges now available, it is easy to find one that fits your needs. Monitoring your activity is a great way to start improving your life. In addition to helping you determine how many calories you're burning per day, trackers can also be used to help keep you accountable.

When you have a particularly lazy day, (we all have them) seeing, "6,553 more steps to go!" can instill a little extra motivation as a reminder that you should have done more today. It can also help you track your improvements in other exercise over time, by tracking the distances and duration of your activities. Whether you invest in a fitness tracker or not, the bottom line is that extra activity is a good idea. Take the opportunity to go for a walk on a nice day, do some yoga, or play with your children or grandchildren. Be aware of what you're doing and try to make smart choices, but be active! Think about your posture as you walk or run, make sure you have relatively new shoes on, and be sure to properly warm up and stretch.

For many people, increased physical activity means

an easier time falling asleep. If you have difficulty falling asleep or staying asleep, try being more active and keep a daily sleep log so you can tell if it's helping.

In addition to physical activity, having a regular bed time can help you fall asleep easier. Your body will become accustomed to your schedule, and know when it is time for sleep. A few minutes of meditation or breathing exercises before bed can also be useful; reading a book just before bed can help your mind relax and allow you to unwind. Try not to spend time in bed unless you intend to be asleep. In other words, don't watch TV, lounge around, or work while in bed. There is conflicting evidence regarding how much sleep you need, so listen to your body. As Dr. Stephanie mentioned, trying to average eight hours is a good benchmark, and you can adjust that based on how you feel. You should be getting enough sleep that you feel energized and refreshed upon waking. If you don't, consider going to bed earlier. If you're regularly active and have a healthy diet, your body may not need as much time to recover as other people.

———————

Though stretching is included in the realm of physical activity, it is also important in regards to your quality of life. Being more flexible will make you less prone to random injuries as you bend and twist throughout the day. There are many different forms of yoga, which build strength and coordination in addition to improving flexibility. You can also stick to plain old stretching! Keep it simple, but be sure to warm up and get stretched out often. If you sit most of the day, get up and walk around, then spend a few minutes stretching out your muscles. When you see your chiropractor, they can help you identify specific stretches that can target the right muscles and ligaments in order to make your spine and core more flexible, reducing your chances of injury.

Making lifestyle changes before visiting a chiro-practor is great – but you should also spend time iden-tifying what you can't do. What specific daily activities, stretches, or sports are you currently unable to do? Make a list of these things, so that as your care progresses you can see your body becoming more capable. It's won-derful to feel like you're getting better, but it's another thing to know it objectively, as you begin shortening the list of things that you can't do.

There was one particular stretch I remember being unable to do. The stretch required me to bend at the waist, reach my arms out in front of me, and slowly rotate them across my body, right to left and then back up again. In the middle I would always hit this one spot where I would lose all strength in my back and it would be nearly impossible to keep my arms stretched out. One day, a few months into my care, I tried the stretch again and couldn't believe I was able to do it without feeling any weakness. It was affirmation to me that I wasn't only feeling better, I was actually getting better. I've found many other things since then that are simi-lar; before care I couldn't do them, and now I am able to do most of them.

Make your list, adding to it as you notice things you almost, but not quite, can do, things you can't do at all, or things you wish you could do better. Your chiropractor might be able to help you identify what is preventing you from achieving these activities, and the care they provide is likely to help you shorten that list.

Becoming complacent is one of the biggest challenges in life. We develop routines that, although helpful for keeping us "busy," end up taking away from our creativity and enjoyment. Make sure that you are spending enough time focusing on yourself, pursuing what matters most to you, and working towards what makes you happy. If you don't enjoy life, Chiropractic care can only do so much for you. But, if you live it for all it is worth, Chiropractic and the environment surrounding it can help you reach new heights. Don't be afraid to try new things and put yourself in the spotlight. You might be amazed at what small changes in your diet, exercise, and mental functioning (less stress) can do in conjunction with Chiropractic. You might even feel like a totally new person!

Appendix B:
What Makes Chiropractic Offices Different?

By Stephanie Foisy Mills, D.C., C.C.W.P.

When comparing Chiropractic offices in your town, you are likely to find that no two are alike. The office is a direct reflection of the doctor's choice of technique (method of adjusting), philosophy of health and healing, and formal education. There are hundreds of different recognized and accepted ways of adjusting the spine; some of these techniques are administered by hand, while others are administered with instruments. Several techniques are considered low force, while others are more physically aggressive. Likewise, there are dozens of different Chiropractic colleges worldwide; each teaches the principles of Chiropractic, but infuses their own unique flavor into the curriculum.

In addition to these differences, the care that you receive in any healthcare environment (Chiropractic included) can be influenced by your insurance benefits. This fact is concerning, and most insurance companies and doctors would rather not talk about it, but it is a reality.

The overall environment in which a doctor chooses to give his adjustments can vary greatly. In this area, it is all about finding what suits you - as a consumer and patient. Are you looking for a peaceful, spa-like experience, or do you gravitate towards a more medical white-coat approach? Maybe you have children and you would rather be in a laid-back, family-friendly atmosphere, where the sounds of children playing aren't considered a nuisance. While it is impossible to cover every variable concerning what makes a Chiropractic practice unique or most suited for your needs, we'll touch on the high points of finding the best-fit practice for you.

Philosophy - Symptoms vs. Health

I would highly recommend locating a Doctor of Chiropractic whose goal is to improve the function and structure of your spine for the long run. Some chiropractors focus solely on your symptoms, such as relieving back pain or headaches. When those symptoms improve, your care is finished. Symptom care only scratches the surface of improving your spine's structure and your overall bodily health. In fact, symptoms can be deceiving; they are often the last thing to show up, and the first thing to leave.

To judge your care solely on how you're feeling is a huge mistake. For example, imagine that your neck took an impact ten years ago in a cheerleading stunt, but you didn't feel any pain at that time. That injury may have caused subluxations that remained silent (no pain) until recent months. You could get adjusted for just a few weeks and have your neck pain disappear. Although the pain is gone, this is *not* a good indicator that a complete healing in the structural shifts of your spine has occurred. Several more weeks or months of specialized care may be necessary to fully heal that old injury, regardless of how great you feel. This is why finding a Doctor of Chiropractic who understands and values creating a healthier spine is key. Be sure you find one that shares in your future goals.

Analysis and Correction

Find a chiropractor who is focused not on your symptoms, but on correcting your subluxations. Key questions to ask are, "How will your care improve the structure of my spine?" and, "How will your care improve my neurological function?" Also ask yourself these questions: Does my chiropractor appear to have a clear method of locating misalignments? Does he have demonstrable ways of assessing my progress, and is he willing to share these results with me? There are hundreds of techniques. As a reference, here is a short list of those focused in the specific correction of subluxation: Chiropractic Biophysics (CBP), Thompson Technique (aka Drop Table), Pettibon, Pierce Results System, Activator Methods, Gonstead, Sacro-Occipital Technique (SOT) and "Upper Cervical Techniques" such as Blair, Toggle Recoil, NUCCA, Atlas Orthogonal, and Grostic.

Insurance

Don't choose a chiropractor simply because he takes your insurance. In fact, you might even want to avoid chiropractors who take your insurance, depending on which plan you belong to. This is because being "in-network" with an insurance company can drastically change the way a chiropractor is expected to practice. In the insurance world, many plans include Chiropractic care on a symptomatic basis.

Wellness care, or care for non-symptomatic subluxations, is not usually covered. Hopefully you already realize that all subluxations (painful or not) are detrimental to your health. Remember, subluxations cause biomechanical issues like arthritis and neurological issues like altered proprioceptive input to the brain - which might not cause pain but which causes harm to the body. You want a chiropractor focused on correcting your entire spine, not simply chasing symptoms in order to receive your insurance company's reimbursement.

Environment

You'll get the most out of your care if you're feeling relaxed and comfortable in your chiropractor's office. Choose a practice where your gut reaction and first impression is an, "uh-huh" and not an, "oh, yikes." You know what I mean. Was the front desk person warm and welcoming? Was the office clean and attractive, or did you look around and want to run for the door?

Don't be surprised to find a "community" adjusting area. The concept of an open treatment area isn't unique to Chiropractic, but it can be a fantastic way to receive your care. It's not only more efficient for you and the doctor, it also allows educational points to benefit everyone in the adjusting area. An open adjusting area also helps assure everyone that there is no inappropriate touching or advances being made. Let's face it, Chiropractic care requires bodily touch and some people are less comfortable with that than others. There's little chance that anything suspicious is happening in a group setting. Open adjusting areas also create a mini-Chiropractic community among practice members, staff, and doctors. This community can add empowerment and facilitate in the healing process itself.

Duration of Normal Office Visit

While this isn't the biggest factor in determining your "best fit" chiropractor, it should be considered. Some Chiropractic techniques only take a few minutes to perform, while others could take 30 minutes, 45 minutes, or more. This doesn't make one better or worse than the other, but if a long visit is going to cause you to feel stressed or pressed for time then it may become an issue. This becomes more concerning if you are expected to attend several office visits per week when you first start your care. In the end this could result in you skipping or rescheduling appointments, which affects the outcome of your care. Be honest with yourself and up front with your practitioner if this is a concern for you.

Other Benefits

When choosing from amongst the chiropractors in your community, you may also want to consider if there are other benefits to being a practice member with a particular office. For example, are there health classes offered in topics like nutrition, stretching, or natural living? Does the chiropractor value healthy lifestyle choices? Are there ways you can stay connected with the practice, like moms' groups, patient events, or social media? Is the doctor easily accessible to you should you have a question or concern?

All of these are key factors in determining the right office, particularly from a doctor's perspective. You now have a better understanding of some of the differences between offices, techniques, and philosophies. In the next chapter, we'll go into more detail about how to go about actually finding the perfect office. For now, start reflecting on what you've learned and try to paint a picture in your mind of what you would like to see in an office that will make it feel less like a doctor's office and more like an extension of your home or community.

APPENDIX C:
FINDING THE RIGHT OFFICE

By Justin C. Chase

Identifying the right Chiropractic office is nothing like playing the lottery; you don't pick one at random and hope you've chosen a winner. Finding the best office begs the question: "What makes an office the best?" The answer to this question is one that will vary among every individual. It requires a clear understanding of your purpose for finding a chiropractor, as well as the ability of the office to assist you in reaching your long term goals. It also includes smaller attributes dictated by your personal taste and aesthetic preferences, such as the feel of the office, the personality of the doctors and staff, the location, et cetera.

Research and Identification

Finding the right clinic begins with the doctors. Do not let yourself be fooled by shiny objects or free services – your pursuit of the right clinic should always begin with the doctor. Potentially knowing little about the medical or Chiropractic fields, how do you identify a good doctor? The answer: Research. You will need to spend time researching and inquiring about the doctors and clinic before making a commitment if you wish to find the best clinic.

Be aware that anywhere a service is being provided, there are always unhappy customers. These customers are usually the most vocal, so don't shy away from an office because of one bad experience, particularly if this bad review is invalidated by a plethora of good ones. In most cases it is fairly easy to search the doctor's name or their practice on the internet and find reviews about the quality of care received there.

While you will not necessarily be able to determine the medical ability of each doctor, that's okay – that is what their college and profession is responsible for. A doctor's reputation is important here, and each chiropractor likely recognizes that. You should be able to determine with minimal effort the reputation of your local office and its practicing doctors. Look for newspaper articles, community involvement, patient reviews and testimonials, as well as the involvement of the doctors in their profession. Can you find articles or information pertaining to Chiropractic on their websites, published in journals or online? Transparency is key – the doctor who wants to educate and inform you is much more likely to be helping you than the doctor who avoids your questions.

It amazes me how many people fail to research their doctors, dentists, surgeons, chiropractors, or athletic trainers. Many people spend more time determining where to get the oil in their car changed. Your doctors hold the quality of your life in their hands. Sure, a bad oil change could cost you a few thousand dollars, but a bad operation or an unprepared doctor could cost you much more than that. I believe that the majority of doctors have your best interests at heart, but in every profession there are those who make poor decisions simply because it is easier, faster, or cheaper. In rare cases, it is because they don't know any better. Do not let yourself be taken advantage of; research your doctors before accepting and paying for care. Not only is this a manner of protection, it can also vastly improve the results you see and feel from your care.

In addition to finding great doctors, you need to make the determination of whether the doctor and their clinic can help you achieve your purpose. What is your purpose? At this point you should have clearly defined long-term goals. How does Chiropractic care fit in with these goals, and how can the doctor and clinic assist you in facilitating them?

If you are looking for a quick fix, then a Chiropractic office that works with insurance companies to provide corrective care may be a good option, as Dr. Stephanie mentioned. This can provide you the opportunity to see what type of difference Chiropractic care can make, while limiting your costs. Once you've seen the benefits of Chiropractic you may find that you want to continue care in an office specializing in wellness care to facilitate the healing process even further and surround yourself with a supportive environment. If, however, your original intention is to maintain long-term care, it would be beneficial to begin your care in a facility offering both corrective care and wellness care. This can provide you with an uninterrupted transition between the two, and help you maintain your relationship with your doctor throughout the process. In many cases you will pay out of pocket, but some insurance companies do offer reimbursement services.

Connecting with Goals

Once you have identified a few doctors or offices for consideration, begin thinking of how they can help support you in the pursuit of your goals. Offices may offer classes at little or no cost for activities such as: yoga, stretching, goal setting, nutrition, core strength, or even meditation. Some will even have health related challenges to keep people engaged and committed. The offerings of your potential offices should be factored in to your final decision.

If you intend to make drastic changes in your life-style over time, perhaps you simply need a Chiropractic office that can offer support. Clinics that offer classes like the ones above are likely knowledgeable in similar areas that can help achieve your goals. It is tough to make lifestyle changes on your own, particularly if you are the first in your circle of friends or family who is trying to make these changes. The support of your Chiropractic office could be the difference between your success and failure. You should be able to find an office with a supportive environment, full of people who will check in with you on your goals and help keep you on track. Your chiropractor has a wealth of knowledge about how the body works – be sure to use every bit of it to your advantage!

If your goals include making simple and small lifestyle changes to achieve better overall health, any Chiropractic office can help. But if you have more intense fitness or nutritional goals, offices that offer classes in these areas could have a lot more to offer you in the long run. By doing your research first, you can ensure that you end up in an office or practice that is capable of supporting you throughout your journey, keeping you motivated and knowledgeable along the way.

Gathering Information

When you go in for your first appointment, you will have paperwork to fill out. Your doctor needs to know all about you in order to protect your investment (your health). You should be prepared to answer standard questions concerning medications that you are on, your insurance care, any surgeries or health problems you've had, and who your primary care doctors are.

While this information is always used to make sure your doctor doesn't recommend or perform something that could be dangerous for you, your chiropractor also wants to know this information in order to see how they can help you. If you're on medication, see a physical therapist, or have other health problems your chiropractor needs to know about them in order to help you. If you hide it from them, they won't be able to provide the information or care you need. Be very transparent with them, as the more informed they are about your needs, the more they can help you learn and grow.

The office may also ask for your interests. Be prepared to discuss your goals, nutrition, fitness levels, and your general lifestyle. Your doctors will be able make recommendations on how you can perform routine tasks, such as driving or using a computer while limiting the effects of these activities on your spine and body. You should also share any goals you have for body changes, such as losing weight, having better posture, or being able to walk without limping. Once again, the more your chiropractor knows about you, the more precise their recommendations can be.

Perhaps the most important information you can provide to your chiropractor is that which relates to accidents, trauma, or stress. Many people are unprepared to provide this, so thinking in advance is crucial. Consider at least the following:

- Have you ever been in a motor vehicle accident? (Include low speed collisions too.)
- Have you ever had a bad fall down stairs, on ice, etc?
- Have you ever broken or fractured a bone, had a dislocated joint, or a bad sprain?
- Do you have history of back pain, neck pain, or injuries?
- Have you ever played collision sports? If so, which ones? Include extreme sports like rafting, hiking, climbing, etc.
- Have you ever been diagnosed with a concussion, or think you've had one that went undiagnosed?
- Are there any repetitive tasks you do every day that tend to cause you pain or discomfort?
- Do you face significant levels of stress at home or at work?

The answers to these questions are absolutely essential for your chiropractor to provide relative care. While they can (and likely will) find the results of these injuries, knowing what to look for will allow them to provide better care. When they find subluxations, knowing this information can help them determine if it was the result of an accident or whether it is a result of your daily routine, helping them make corrective recommendations for you.

The last major question you should be prepared to answer is, "Why are you seeking care?" In order to best serve you, your chiropractor needs to know what you think is most important concerning your visits. It will allow them to tailor their services to your needs. Be sure to let them know if your goals change too – in just a short conversation with a chiropractor, your goals may change from relieving pain to gaining overall health and limiting the number of medications you have to take to stay healthy.

This is a lot of information. Be prepared to answer all these questions so that your first visit is one full of answers! The more you've thought about your reasons for coming, the more your chiropractor will be able to explain to you. They can help you understand how the care you'll receive from them can help you reduce or eliminate many of the symptoms you feel. Unlike medication, Chiropractic is aimed at correcting and treating the causes of your ills, not simply covering up or treating the effects.

Asking Your Own Questions

While your chiropractor needs to know information about you, you are surely going to have questions of your own. This book is intended to help answer many of your questions prior to ever visiting an office, but you'll probably want to know even more by the time you meet a doctor. Don't be afraid to ask questions! It is very likely that you will want to know more about what your chiropractor plans to do to you. They should be happy to answer your questions about the type of Chiropractic adjustments they use, and help you understand what you should expect.

After the doctor reviews your file and sees your medical history, you may want to ask what they think they can do to help you. They will be able to provide you with information about what they're looking for, and explain what they're going to do to fix it once they find it. Your first appointment is one of many opportunities to better understand your care. You can also ask questions about your chiropractor's knowledge of the other joints in the body, since they can check or adjust those for you, too.

Is it okay to ask about their schooling? I don't think it's inappropriate to ask a doctor about the knowledge they possess. You are putting the care of your body in their hands – the least they can do is make sure you are comfortable and confident in their ability to take care of you. Asking questions about their knowledge and experience can help you build a relationship full of trust with your doctor.

It is also perfectly acceptable to ask your doctor what the next step is. Particularly if this is your first experience with Chiropractic, you may not have any idea how it all works! Ask about the process, so that you can understand how the office works, what steps are going to be taken to get you into care, and if there is anything else you should know. This is also a good time to ask about any other services the clinic offers, such as classes, training, or other activities if you haven't already done so.

In short, when it comes to finding the right office and preparing for your first appointment, you should to do three things: research, prepare your health history, and think about what you want to learn. If you research an office and find one with a good reputation, great doctors, or a big presence in the community, go on in and talk to them. Check out the atmosphere and get a feel for what the office has to offer.

Once you've picked an office or narrowed it down, get your health history ready. Consider all the questions mentioned above, and even ask your parents or siblings if you had any accidents when you were a child. The more information you have, the better. When you have your history covered start thinking about what you want to learn from your chiropractor.

When you are ready, go in and make an appointment! Ask if there are any specials on pricing for first appointments, and be sure to tell your office if a friend referred you to them. Now that you're prepared with information and questions, what does your chiropractor plan to do at the first appointment? Dr. Stephanie discusses that next, so keep reading!

APPENDIX D:
THE FIRST
APPOINTMENT

By Stephanie Foisy Mills, D.C., C.C.W.P.

First off: don't arrive at your first visit expecting an adjustment. This could lead to disappointment should the chiropractor require an examination or other testing before beginning care (and they should). Your doctor's intention with the first visit is to create a doctor–patient relationship, examine your spine, and be available to clarify any questions you may have leading up to care.

The key question they want to answer is: are there any subluxations in your spine? Most chiropractors will ask questions about your health history, any present or chronic health concerns, and seek to gain an understanding of traumas and stresses that could have contributed to shifts in your spine. The chiropractor should also evaluate your spinal alignment through palpating (feeling) your vertebrae for alignment and/or motion. This is the bare minimum. There are dozens of other methods of assessing the neuro–structural function of your spine, some of which will be used by your doctor depending on their chosen Chiropractic technique.

Postural assessment and range of motion testing can give an understanding of shifts in your spine and can be used to objectively quantify your progress during a course of care. Specialized equipment to detect variations in skin temperature can be used to locate a subluxation and monitor progress as well. Prone and supine leg check analysis can give information about neurological involvement and the location and direction of any present misalignments. Some doctors perform muscle testing or a more traditional muscle strength and reflex test. Many doctors who specialize in structural correction rely heavily on radiographs (x-rays) as a key part of their assessment.

The methods your chiropractor utilizes to detect and locate vertebral subluxations is specific to their chosen technique. Just remember, a skilled doctor will have a system of analysis and will utilize it at all times during clinical decision making. Beware of the doctor who welcomes you into his practice, barely says, "Hello!" and ushers you onto his table to be manipulated without a proper exam.

A quick fix or "cracking" by a doctor will short change you on the larger benefits of Chiropractic adjustments, such as the correction of spinal shifts and the resolution of neurological compromises. While it is possible for some doctors to do all of their testing, analysis, and information synthesis on your first visit and also deliver an adjustment that same day, many doctors will require more time. Don't be put off by having to wait to receive your first adjustment. It's a sign that your doctor cares and wants to deliver the best care to you based on their education, technique, and philosophy.

Before you choose to have your first adjustment, your doctor should explain what they have found. After this discussion, you should have a strong understanding of your problem areas, and how they relate to your health. You should also have an idea about the long-term outlook of your case and care, both in prognosis and cost. In other words, your doctor should take the time to sit down with you, review the findings of your examination and explain his planned approach for improving your spinal condition. They'll cover how frequently you should come in, and for how long, as well as the associated costs with this approach. Know that these may change depending on how your body reacts, but they can be used as a general guideline.

If your chiropractor recommends only a few visits to help you feel better, take pause and let them know you are looking for more than a quick fix. If you've read this far into our book, you're likely fully invested in rebuilding your health – the right way. Don't be afraid to explain this to your doctor. They should reach beyond symptoms and outline a plan for correcting the shifts in your spine and any associated neurological dysfunction.

Be sure that he or she has a clear way of measuring progress over the next several weeks and months. This will help both of you track your progress over the course of your care. In most cases, your doctor should help you develop a solid plan for stretching and exercise, as well as provide advice on how to best nourish your body. These steps, among others, are warranted and make a good complement to your Chiropractic adjustments.

Communication is the key component of a successful doctor-patient relationship. Be forthcoming on your first visit when sharing your history. During the report of the doctor's examination findings, engage in the conversation about your condition, and share your short-term and long-term health goals. If you have a spouse or significant other who can support you on this journey, bring them along to your follow-up appointment.

Remember that this is your time with the doctor, so make the most of it, and don't be afraid to ask questions!

APPENDIX E:
WHAT HAPPENS NOW?

By Justin C. Chase

After you have started receiving Chiropractic adjustments, you might wonder, "What happens now?" The answer is one that is different for everyone. Some people will notice a change in the way their body feels and functions immediately, while for others it may change at a slow pace over time. Don't be discouraged if after your initial adjustment you feel discomfort or pain; healing is not always enjoyable at first. When you break a bone or dislocate a joint, the first steps in the healing process can be extremely painful, but in the end the result is worth it.

Your chiropractor is going to be your most valuable asset in this part of the process, so be sure to communicate with him about how you're feeling. He may be able to make the process more bearable, or help you understand what is happening to your body in greater detail. Your body may resist change, even if it is change that will be helpful to it in the long run.

Your chiropractor's job is to ensure you are getting the treatment your body needs. He is going to use all of his knowledge, and make use of the tools at his disposal to monitor your progress. By communicating effectively with your chiropractor, you can make sure that you are both on the same page. Regardless of how your body initially responds to care, there are a number of things you can do to help facilitate the process.

We have discussed in some depth the importance of physical activity, stretching, and nutrition throughout this book. Those should remain in the forefront of your lifestyle changes as you continue throughout, but there are other things you can do to help facilitate your care. Though I just spoke of communicating your concerns to your doctor, understand that communication is a two-way street. Just as your feedback is important to your doctor, his feedback should be equally as important to you.

Don't be afraid to ask questions when he presents you with information you may not understand completely. When he reviews your progress, ask questions! Was there a lot of progress? If not, what can you do to help? If there was, what might you have been doing to facilitate it that you should continue doing? The more information you have about your care, the better informed your decisions will be every day. By communicating each time you visit your chiropractor, you can help identify the choices you are making that are helping or harming your care.

If you make a lifestyle change like increasing daily activity, stretching before bed, using a standing workstation, etc. - ask your doctor for feedback to help you determine if these changes are having a positive effect! If you don't ask, you'll likely never know for sure.

Your chiropractor may also assign you specific exercises or tasks to help your body make the necessary adjustments. Your commitment to performing these tasks is essential to getting the best care possible. If your chiropractor didn't believe they would help, he wouldn't be asking you to do them. Demonstrate how important your body is to you by following his instructions on technique and frequency for any and all tasks assigned. Don't forget to ask what the activities are for and how they'll help you! A proper explanation may give you some extra motivation when you really don't think you can make the time to do it. Knowing the consequences of inaction is every bit as significant as knowing the positive consequences that are associated with performing the activity as you are directed.

If you want to recover your health as quickly as possible, follow your doctor's recommendations. Most of the activities he assigns you will have little or no cost, yet still carry with them the potential for significant benefits to your body.

You may also find that some chiropractors recommend massage therapy in conjunction with Chiropractic care. There have been studies conducted fairly recently to support the use of massage therapy in treating low back pain, as well as joint pain from arthritis (Burkhart, 2014). Though massage therapy has been in existence for a long period of time, there is great difficulty performing studies with such a hands on treatment – there has not been an effective placebo to simulate the experience of a massage, so most studies remain inconclusive or only partially answer the questions at hand. In theory, muscle and soft tissue memory is one of the primary reasons that the body takes time to begin holding Chiropractic adjustments. After adjustments are made, muscles initially resist the change, limiting the length of time that the body can hold the adjustment. By combining Chiropractic care with massage therapy, muscles are more relaxed and thus are less likely to resist the changes being made by your chiropractor. Even if adding massage therapy to your regular repertoire of care does not directly influence the results of your Chiropractic care, it still carries the benefits of massage therapy. Your muscles and body can feel more relaxed, and the mental effects of a massage can help relieve the stress we experience in our lives.

If you followed our recommendations earlier in this book, you will have started a log or journal to keep track of activities that you were unable to perform in the past. Be sure to review this frequently, and make additional notes in relation to your progress. You can also keep a log of how you feel physically and mentally on a daily basis, to help you identify how your care is affecting the way you feel. Make note of how well you sleep, how any changes you have made affected your well-being, and in general just make notes concerning your overall health. Pay attention to how long it takes you to recover from sickness, and even make notes of how well your body held adjustments (from your chiropractor's feedback).

To help maximize the benefits of your care, avoid missing Chiropractic visits. If you feel you need to make extra visits, do so - particularly if you're feeling a sickness coming on or are trying to recover from an injury. The same applies if you spent a day doing heavy lifting or any kind of serious physical exertion. Just don't

miss your appointments. The reason visits are sched-
uled more frequently during initial care is that the body
needs constant, small "nudges" in the right direction.
Skipping a visit is like cancelling a training session for
a marathon. One missed appointment might not make
a huge impact, but if it becomes a frequent occurrence
it can significantly limit the effects of the training your
body is getting from your chiropractor. Remember that
you really are training for a marathon – it's called life,
and it waits for no one. Be sure your priorities are in
order when you have a conflict in your scheduling, and
do your best to make up your appointments if you find
you do have to cancel them.

Our focus now shifts to the choices that we make on
a daily basis. At this point, with what you have learned
throughout your reading and in conjunction with your
chosen Chiropractic office, you should be more informed
than ever before about how the choices you make impact
your life. This newfound knowledge will allow you to be
proactive, and weigh your options at each crossroads.

Most people only make adjustments when confront-
ed with pain or discomfort – this is called being reac-
tive. As you progress in your care you should become
proactive. Thinking about potential situations and how
best to handle them will prepare you to act appropriately when the time comes. This applies to routine tasks,
as well as those we seldom encounter. When emptying
the dishwasher for example, have you ever considered
the way you bend over to reach for the dishes? Do you
bend at the waist, or do you round out your back as you
reach down? When you wear a backpack, do you carry
more than you need, putting excess strain on your back,

neck, and shoulders? These are the little things that can make our lives more difficult, unless we choose to think about them and find better solutions.

This is your opportunity to put what you have learned to good use and make smart choices. Essentially if you are sitting, bending, twisting, or carrying weight, you should be carefully considering how you complete these processes. Make sure that each thing you sit on supports you in the correct way, helping you to maintain good posture. Put in the time to make sure that your seat is properly adjusted in your car, that you are using the right chair at work, and that you are lightly engaging your core whenever you are sitting.

When you bend, bend at the waist, not at the back. Bend your legs when possible, and try to avoid hanging your neck and head out in front of your body. Whenever you twist make sure your feet pivot with your body, that your core is engaged and supportive, and that you don't end up in an awkward, uncomfortable position.

If you're carrying weight, make sure it is evenly distributed. Carry groceries with both hands, don't sling your gym bag across your body, and buy backpacks that offer adequate support. Don't forget to buy new shoes, either. Wearing worn out shoes, or ones that offer poor support can affect not only our feet and ankles, but our knees, pelvis, and overall posture. Each of these small actions, when performed improperly, take away from your health in both the short term and the long term. We only have one body – we need to take care of it to ensure it lasts us a lifetime.

In addition to how we do things, we need to consider *what* we do. Are we making decisions about what we should and shouldn't be doing? For example, I love tubing behind the boat in the summer at the lake with my cousins. But I have now become aware of the damage it does to my neck and spine. Although it is a blast to do, the fifteen minutes of enjoyment does not outweigh the pain I feel for days. We need to carefully examine each activity we do, and determine whether the benefits outweigh the other consequences.

Is it really so important to do something you know is going to hurt you? When we decide that an activity is worth the risk, we can take steps to minimize the damage that is done. If we are doing something that puts excess strain on our neck or back, we can make sure we adequately strengthen the areas involved, and spend time increasing their flexibility and range of motion. Spend the time weighing your options, and make conscious choices in regards to your health. This process can be the difference between a future we can enjoy, and a future full of regrets.

What is the most important thing you can do in regards to maintaining and improving the care you receive from your chiropractor? Use your brain.

You have been informed, you have been advised, and you have had the opportunity to determine your goals and reasons for seeking care. Now use your mind, and make smart choices. Help yourself, by examining the way that you live your life, how you treat your body, and how you want your future to look. Use your resources to continue learning.

You have the power to set the course of your life. Use that power consciously – don't pretend something isn't hurting you when you know it is. Instead, make the tougher choice and do what is right. Either stop doing what you are doing, or find a way to do it better. If you can improve on one task every single day, you will be amazed at the difference it can make in your life. This is something you can live by.

It doesn't matter if you are sweeping the floor, or running a marathon. Find a way to do it better, faster, and more effectively. Limit the damage it causes, and maximize the good it brings to your life. You control your future, and only you can decide whether you will help yourself, or whether you will continuing treating effects rather than their underlying causes. Make the hard choice and take care of yourself, because no one else is going to do it for you.

RESOURCES:
COMPLETE REFERENCE
LIST

Alcantara, J., Davis, A., & Oman, R. E. (2009). The effects of Chiropractic on a child with transient motor tics using Gonstead & Toggle Techniques. Journal of Pediatric, Maternal & Family Health - Chiropractic(2), 1-9.

Arsenault, D., Johnson, K., King, H., Lockwood, M., Quist, R., & Tettambel, M. (2003, December). Ostepathic manipulative treatment in prenatal care: A retrospective case control design study. Journal of the American Osteopathic Association, 103, 577-582.

Banks, E., Bauman, A., Chey, T., Korda, R. J., & van der Ploeg, H. P. (2012). Sitting time and all-cause mortality risk in 222,297 Australian adults. Archives of Internal Medicine, 494-500. doi:10.1001/archinternmed.2011.2174

Buckley, T., Fethney, J., Hanson, P. S., Shaw, E., Tofler, G. H., & Y Soo Hoo, S. (2015). Triggering of Acute Coronary Occlusion by episodes of anger. European Heart Journal: Acute Cardiovascular Care, 1-6.

Cambron, J. A., Sarnat, R. L., & Winterstein, J. (2007, May). Clinical utilization and cost outcomes from an integrative medicine independent physician association: An additional three year update. Journal of Manipulative and Physiological Therapeutics, 30(4), 263-269.

Deaths and Mortality. (2015, January 20). Retrieved from Center for Disease Control and Prevention: http://www.cdc.gov/nchs/fastats/deaths.htm

Elster, E. (2003). Upper cervical Chiropractic care for a nine-year-old male with Tourette Syndrome, Attention Deficit Hyperactivity Disorder, Depression, Asthma, Insomnia, and headaches: A case report. Journal of Vertebral Subluxation Research, 1-11.

Elster, E. (2003). Upper cervical Chiropractic care for a patient with chronic migraine headaches with an appendix summarizing an additional 100 headache cases. Journal of Vertebral Subluxation Research, 1-10.

Esch, S. (1988). Newborn with atlas subluxation/absent rooting reflex from case reports in Chiropractic Pediatrics. ACA Journal of Chiropractic.

Fallon, J. M. (1994). Textbook on Chiropractic & pregnancy. Arlington, Virginia: International Chiropractic Association.

Flesia, J. M. (1992, March). The vertebral subluxation complex: An integrative perspective. International Review of Chiropractic, 25-27.

Haavik, H. (2014). The reality check: A quest to understand Chiropractic from the inside out. Auckland, New Zealand: Haavik Research Limited.

Hansraj, K. K. (2014). Assessment of stresses in the cervical spine caused by posture and position of the head. Surgical Technology International(XXV), 277-279.

Homewood, A. E. (1973). The neurodynamics of the vertebral subluxation. (2 ed.). Canada: Chiropractic Publishers.

Lathrop, J. M., & Yoshimura, R. (2015, May). Improvement in sensory modulation & functional disorders in a female pediatric patient undergoing Chiropractic care. Annals of Vertebral Subluxation Research, 108-118.

Lauro, A., & Mouch, B. (1991). Chiropractic effects on athletic ability. The Journal of Chiropractic Research and Clinical Investigation, 84-87.

Manello, D., Rupert, R. L., & Sandefur, R. (2000). Maintenance care: Health promotion services administered to US Chiropractic patients ages 65 and older, part II. Journal of Manipulative and Physiological Therapeutics, 23(1), 10-19.

Nilsson, N., Nordsteen, J., & Wiberg, J. (1999, October). The short-term effect of spinal manipulation in the treatment of Infantile Colic: A randomized controlled clinical trial with a blinded observer. Journal of Manipulative Physiological Therapeutics, 517-522.

Pistolese, R. A. (2002). The Webster Technique: a Chiropractic technique with obstetric implications. Journal of Manipulative Physiological Therapeutics, E1-E9.

Shaw, G. (2003). When to adjust: Chiropractic and pregnancy. Journal of American Chiropractic Association, 8-16.

Sharpless, S. K. (1975). Susceptibility of spinal roots to compression block. National Institute of Health, Research Status of Spinal Manipulative Therapy. DHEW Publications 76-998:155.

Windwer, S., & Wolfman, M. (2015, April). Efficacy of Chiropractic adjustments versus self-manipulation of the lumbar spine in a 17-year-old male with chronic low back pain: A case study. Annals of Vertebral Subluxation Research, 43-47.

ADDITIONAL RESOURCE LIST

Books

Chicken Soup for the Chiropractic Soul by Jack Canfield and Mark Victor Hansen

Chiropractic Works: Adjusting to a Higher Quality of Life by Timothy J. Feuling

Everyday Paleo by Sarah Fragoso and Robb Wolf

Impossible Cure: The Promise of Homeopathy by Amy L. Lansky

Love Your Body: Your Path to Transformation, Health, and Healing by N. D. Barry Taylor

Our Daily Meds: How the Pharmaceutical Companies Transformed Themselves into Slick Marketing Machines and Hooked the Nation on Prescription Drugs by Melody Petersen

Overdosed America: The Broken Promise of American Medicine by John Abramson

Seeds of Deception: Exposing Industry and Government Lies about the Safety of the Genetically Engineered Foods You're Eating by Jeffrey M. Smith

The 14 Foundational Premises for Scientific and Philosophical Validation of the Chiropractic Wellness Paradigm by James L. Chestnut

The Reality Check by Heidi Haavik

The Wellness and Prevention Paradigm by James L. Chestnut

Documentaries

Food, Inc. directed by Robert Kenner

Generation RX directed by Kevin P. Miller

The Beautiful Truth: The World's Simplest Cure for Cancer directed by Steve Kroschel

Websites

http://www.heidihaavik.com
http://www.icpa4kids.org/
http://robbwolf.com/what-is-the-paleo-diet/
http://www.nvic.org/
http://www.holisticmoms.org/
http://www.vertebralsubluxation.org/

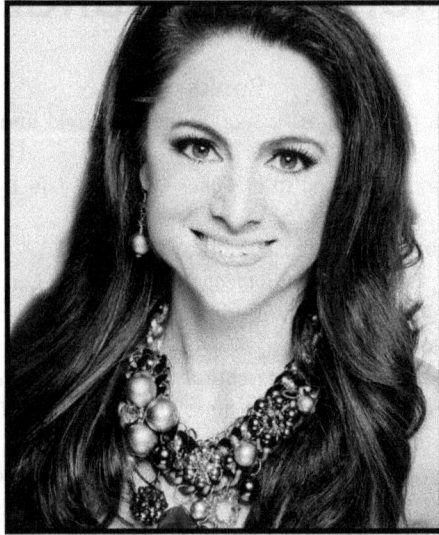

Dr. Stephanie Mills is a Presidential Scholar and Summa cum Laude graduate of Palmer College of Chiropractic. She was the first chiropractor in her state to receive the Certified Chiropractic Wellness Practitioner (C.C.W.P.) distinction from the International Chiropractic Association and is also an ICPA practitioner with Webster Technique certification. Dr. Stephanie hosts a weekly radio show in New Hampshire on WTPL 107.7 FM to promote Chiropractic, vitalistic principles, and healthy lifestyle choices. In addition, she is a nationally recognized and sought-after speaker on numerous health topics. Her most important role, though, is "Mom" to two well-adjusted daughters, Brooke and Emilee.

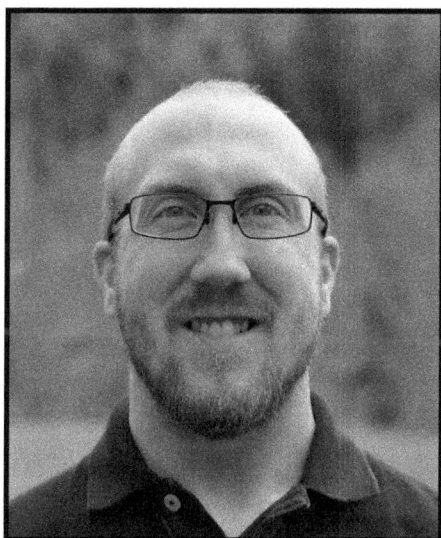

Justin C. Chase is a small business owner, writer, tutor, and certified Secondary Mathematics Educator in New Hampshire. He is also a graduate student enrolled in a Master of Leadership program at Granite State College. He uses his coaching skills to help individuals of all ages gain perspective on topics by encouraging them to examine all angles and search for answers to the right questions. Justin intends to continue developing his business by writing and publishing resources on controversial topics in the Health, Leadership, and Education fields. Always learning new things, Justin enjoys staying current on business, philosophy, and technology. When he is not working, Justin likes to spend time with family, reading, staying fit, and working on automotive projects.